LIVING WITH ENDOMETRIOSIS

A practical guide to the causes and treatments

Caroline Hawkridge

Illustrated by
Karen Huckvale

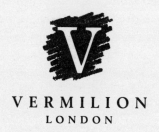

VERMILION
LONDON

First published by Macdonald Optima in 1989

1 3 5 7 9 10 8 6 4 2

This revised edition published in the United Kingdom in 1996 by Vermilion an imprint of Ebury Press
Random House UK Ltd
Random House
20 Vauxhall Bridge Road
London SW1V 2SA

Random House Australia (Pty) Ltd
20 Alfred Street, Milsons Point, Sydney,
New South Wales 2061, Australia

Random House New Zealand Limited
18 Poland Road, Glenfield,
Auckland 10, New Zealand

Random House, South Africa (Pty) Limited
PO Box 337, Bergvlei, South Africa

Random House UK Limited Reg. No. 954009

A CIP catalogue record for this book is available from the British Library.

ISBN 0 09 181261 5

Typeset in Sabon by Deltatype Ltd, Ellesmere Port, Cheshire
Printed and bound in Great Britain by Mackays of Chatham, plc

Papers used by Vermilion are natural, recyclable products made from wood grown in sustainable forests.

CONTENTS

*The first edition of this book was dedicated to
Ailsa Irving, who founded the
Endometriosis Society in 1981,
and my parents.
This second edition is for Graham.*

ACKNOWLEDGMENTS

I was very moved recently when Imogen Bertin e-mailed me from Ireland to tell me how she'd discovered 400 women with endometriosis supporting each other in cyberspace. I realised how much the world had changed since 1981 when I met a small self-help group in London which became the Endomentriosis Society and even since the first edition of this book was published. But I also realised how much remains the same. Women with endometriosis still need information, support and friendship with each other whether it is in cyberspace, self-help groups or through the pages of a book.

Another moving aspect of up-dating this book was discovering the huge increase in endometriosis research in the last five years. However, this did add to my task and I'm grateful to Helen Alexander, Jane Hawkridge, Dr Anne Hawkridge, Dr Sean Hughes, Lhyn Norman and Graham Oakes for their assistance. I'd also like to thank Imogen Bertin for her information on WISTENDO and her willingness to help women access the Internet.

My gratitude to all the women who wrote their stories for the first edition remains. Their voices still lift off the pages after all this time. Dr Stephen Kennedy and David Hawkridge provided enthusiastic support and advice for the original manuscript and various members of the Endometriosis Society commented. Karen Huckvale and I developed the illustrations. Nicky Wesson and Lesley Misrahi (formerly Mabbett) contributed the original Chapters 7 and 8 and 9 respectively. Lesley did most of the up-dating of Chapter 8.

My thanks remain to the Endometriosis Society for making the original survey of 800 members possible. I designed the survey, Sharon Fordham and Roy Evans worked on the questionnaires and Indal Ltd generously gave us free computing

CONTENTS

facilities. The results were presented in a communication libre at the First International Symposium on endometriosis in France, 1987.

I'm also grateful to my commissioning editor, Harriet Griffey, who backed this book before most people had heard of endometriosis and my current editor, Sarah Sutton, who has continued to back this book now it is one of many.

Cheshire, 1995

FOREWORD

'There is little worse in life than the misery of trying to endure intractable pain or prolonged infertility'. These were the opening words that I wrote in 1988 to the Foreword of the first edition of Understanding Endometriosis. It would have been marvellous to commence the Foreword to this edition with the words 'There have been enormous advances in our understanding of endometriosis since Caroline's book was first published, which have resulted in better ways of diagnosing the condition and more effective treatments'. Sadly, it is not possible to make such a statement because in these 8 years, our knowledge of the condition has advanced very little. In fact, we probably know less now about endometriosis than we ever have because the results of recent research have provided us with such confusing results.

Whatever the state of our scientific knowledge, the human tragedy of this chronic condition perisists and I am as troubled now as I was 8 years ago on hearing that many endometriosis sufferers endure their symptoms with little support. Life for many of the women who have contributed to this book has become unbearable and their tragedy is compounded by the realisation that there is no magical cure for their symptoms.

Most of us have an expectation, which is not unreasonable at the end of the 20th century, that when we describe a set of symptoms to a doctor, the doctor will not only be able to diagnose what is wrong but he/she will also be able to get rid of the symptoms. On reading these pages, it is clear to me that conventional medicine often fails to meet the expectations of women with pelvic pain. Until we understand what causes endometriosis, sufferers must realise that the treatments we offer may only be palliative and may not work. Consequently, it is often necessary to turn to alternative strategies and therapies to improve a woman's quality of life and the need is greater than ever for self-help groups, such as the Endometriosis Society, to provide relief simply by giving sufferers the opportunity to share their experiences.

The book explains medical facts in an easily understandable way. It offers an up-to-date account of modern research and discusses the progress that has been made in the treatment of infertility through the use of assisted reproduction techniques, such as in vitro fertilisation. It will provide some much needed hope to couples who long for a child, by recounting accounts of successful IVF treatment in women, for whom the idea of pregnancy previously seemed a remote possibility. It considers alternative forms of therapy and some of the wider issues of being an endometriosis sufferer that are frequently ignored by the medical profession such as the effect of the condition upon the psyche and inter-personal relationships. More than anything else the book vividly describes what it can feel like to be burdened with a chronic disease: to cope with such emotions as the disappointment of failed therapy or disease recurrence; to suffer in silence the agony of painful periods and painful intercourse; to undergo the stress of infertility investigations and treatments.

A recurrent theme throughout the book is the anger that many women feel at the way they have been treated by the medical system and by society at large. I hope that this book will help to narrow the gap between some endometriosis sufferers and their doctors. It will demonstrate to sufferers some of the difficulties inherent in making an accurate diagnosis and in treating the condition. It will also serve to remind us as doctors just how debilitating endometriosis can be.

Sadly, despite years of research, we still do not understand the cause of endometriosis nor why it should cause symptoms. Many researchers are sceptical about the theory that it arises becuse of some disturbance in the normal processes occuring in the peritoneal cavity which allow endometrial cells to implant in some women and not in others. Therefore, the theory that endometriosis is caused by an immunological deficiency remains to be proven.

The research we are currently performing in Oxford, in

collaboration with major research centres throughout the world, aims to identify a gene or set of genes that is responsible for conferring susceptibility to endometriosis. We suspect that a woman's predisposition to develop endometriosis is genetically determined, but that additional factors are required to initiate the development of the disease such as heavy, frequent periods or possibly even environmental agents such as dioxins. The identification of the genetic determinants of endometriosis should allow us to understand better the causes of the disease. Based upon this knowledge, we may in time also be able to develop more effective forms of treatment and ways of making a diagnosis without the use of laparoscopy.

Dr Stephen Kennedy is a Senior Research Fellow in Reproductive Medicine in the Nuffield Department of and Gynaecology at the University of Oxford and an Honorary Consultant at The Women's Centre, John Radcliffe Hospital, Oxford.

1
UNDERSTANDING YOUR BODY

Understanding endometriosis and its treatment is easier if you can imagine what you are like inside and how the menstrual cycle works. Understanding your body can be fun – and you don't need to be Einstein to get the basic idea!

HOW YOU ARE ARRANGED

Have you ever wondered how far apart your ovaries are? Or how big your uterus is? Or even what an ovary is like? Or how the menstrual cycle always happens in the right order over and over again?

A textbook chapter on the female menstrual cycle usually

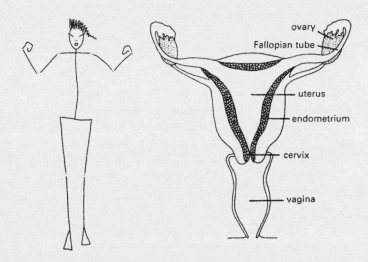

Getting to know your anatomy: front view.

starts with a diagram in which the uterus is seen from the front with the fallopian tubes and ovaries sttetched out on either side. Although this may be a convenient way to look at it in textbooks, it does not really help women to understand themselves. In reality the Fallopian tubes and ovaries are often tucked behind the uterus, which leans forward. The difference is much easier to imagine if you think of youself standing upright with your arms ourstretched, fists clenched into ovaries, as in the first diagram. To change to the position in the second diagram, bend forward at the waist and curve your arms behind your back near your sides.

Imagine yourself as a soft and floppy uterus from the waist up and that you are resting on the bladder which sits snugly in front of you while the bowel comes down behind you. The uterus tends to slide into different positions depending on how full the bladder and the bowel are. The uterus iself is about the size of your fist and each ovary is like a walnut.

If you imitate the uterus position shown in the second illustration you can feel your back muscles holding your body's weight as it leans forward. Similarly, your uterus also needs a means of support. The best way to understand this is to clench

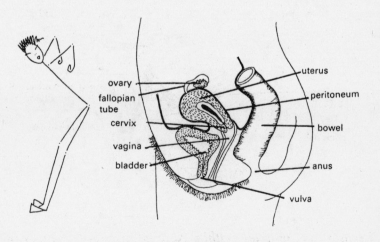

Getting to know your anatomy: side view.

your pelvic floor muscles. If you are not sure how to do this, try the following next time you need to urinate. Sitting with your legs apart, stop the flow of urine in midstream and notice which muscles you use to do it. When you have got the feel of it, try it again later when you are not on the toilet – you can do it sitting down in the office or driving, standing up ironing or waiting at a bus stop. No one can tell! The muscles you are using are known as the levator ani muscles, although most people simply refer to them as the pelvic floor muscles.

The uterus is also supported by bands of elastic tissue known as the cardinal ligaments or transverse cervical ligaments. Some diagrams of the uterus show the round ligament and broad ligament instead, although they are not very important. The round ligament is only a weak 'guy-rope' which is tightened to move the uterus forward. The broad ligament is not a ligament at all; it is a fold of peritoneum, the membrane lining the abdomen, and is easiest to imagine as a 'poncho' of fibrous tissue hanging over the uterus, with the ovaries like hands sticking out of the sleeves.

At this stage you might wonder why your uterus flops forward at all. It is not a stupid question. Think of the lower half of your body as a bucket, with the bottom taken out and replaced by a

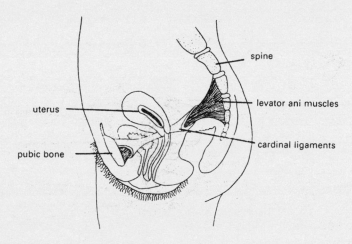

Levator ani muscles within cardinal ligaments supporting uterus.

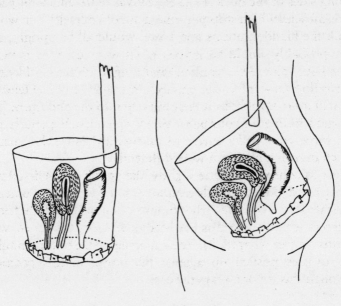

Understanding the pelvic tilt.

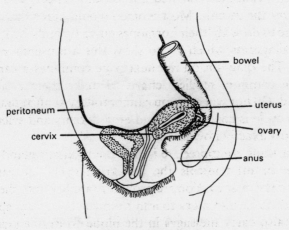

Retroverted uterus.

piece of canvas. The bones in your pelvic girdle are like the strong sides of the bucket and the canvas represents your pelvic floor muscles which stop you falling out of yourself! You would think the bladder, uterus and bowel would all be upright, and they probably would be if your pelvis was not tilted forward from your spine. As a result of this tilting, both the bladder and uterus flop forward under gravity, although the bowel tends to be held more upright as it continues up into the abdomen. You can get a feeling for your pelvic tilt by walking in high heels; this will force your pelvic girdle to tip forward more than usual, which in turn makes you walk differently.

Just to confuse the issue slightly, the uterus can be fixed in a 'retroverted' position. This is quite common amongst women in general, but is particularly common amongst endometriosis sufferers where the uterus has become stuck to the bowel with scar tissue (see Chapter 2). You can imagine the fallopian tubes and ovaries pushed up against the bowel in this position, although this is not always the case.

YOUR MENSTRUAL CYCLE

You are the expert on your own pattern of bodily changes during the menstrual cycle. You may have used charts to record your periods, your ovulation, and changes such as breast tenderness, irritability, bloatedness or differences in sexual feelings over the month. Most women would agree that these changes are to do with 'their hormones going up and down', but textbook diagrams which try to show this are usually rather daunting. The diagram on the next page combines a cartoon with some common medical charts to make them easier to understand. Do not worry if you cannot follow at all at first; the menstrual cycle is complicated and even doctors and scientists do not know exactly how it works.

The first thing to appreciate is that the pituitary gland (just below the brain) controls the menstrual cycle by sending messages to the ovaries. You are probably familiar with the idea of nerves carrying messages to and from the brain, but special chemicals also carry messages in the blood from one place to another. These chemicals are called hormones.

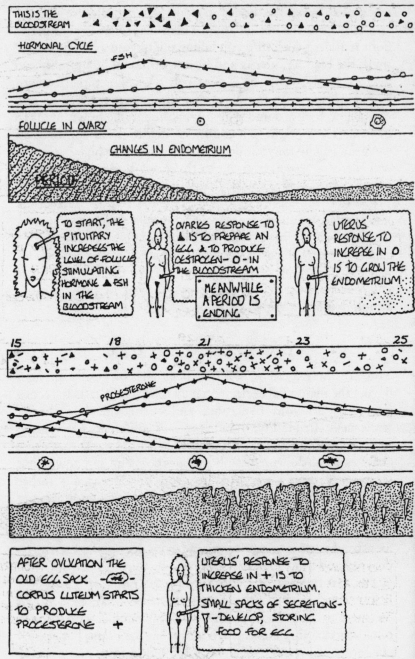

What happens in your menstrual cycle.

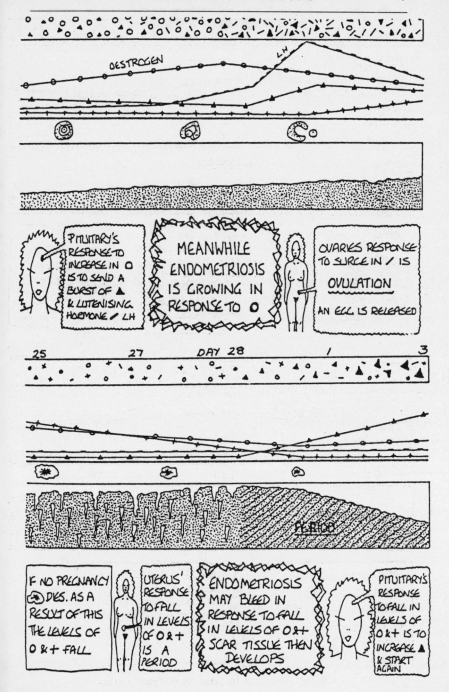

How hormones work

The way hormones work is easier to understand if you bear in mind a few simple ideas. Nerves tend to be like light switches; what happens will depend on whether they are on or off. Hormones are more like sounds since they can be on at different levels, so more varied and complicated messages can be sent. Organs such as the ovaries and the uterus are programmed to react in their own way to a change in the level of 'loudness' of a hormone circulating in the bloodstream.

Hormones and the menstrual cycle

The diagram on pages 6 and 7 illustrates how hormone levels change in a set pattern every mentstrual cycle. Since the menstrual cycle repeats itself, you can start to look at what happens at any stage, but day 1 is usually counted as the first day of your period, with menstrual bleeding usually ending between days 4 and 7. Early in the cycle the pituitary gland releases more follicle stimulating hormone (FSH) into the bloodstream. One or other ovary will respond when FSH gets to a certain level. As its name suggests, this hormone stimulates a group of ovarian cells called a follicle to prepare an egg. At this stage the ovary starts to produce the hormone oestrogen.

Rising oestrogen levels mean different things to different organs. The uterus reacts by growing the lining (known as endometrium) to receive the egg, if it becomes fertilised. To the pituitary gland, the rise signals that an egg is being developed and it is time to send a burst of luteinising hormone (LH) into the bloodstream.

The LH surge causes the follicle to release the egg (ovulation). Ovulation occurs around day 14, although this varies from woman to woman and may not be regular for the same person. It usually happens about two weeks before a period starts, so women with longer cycles also ovulate later. You can find out when you are ovulating by making a temperature chart. Ask at your local family planning clinic or GP surgery.

Once ovulation has taken place, the follicle turns yellow and is then known as the corpus luteum – translated as yellow body. The corpus luteum produces another hormone called progeste-rone, to make sure the endometrium – the lining of the uterus –

is ready to receive the egg. Textbooks say progesterone makes the endometrium secretory; little sacks of secretions develop which store food for the egg. If the egg is fertilised, it will plant itself into the endometrium and release its own hormone, human chorionic gonadotrophin (hCG), to make sure the body continues to look after it. Pregnancy tests are designed to detect small amounts of hCG that appear in your urine.

Unless there is a pregnancy, the corpus luteum only lives for a short time. As it regresses, the progesterone and oestrogen levels fall, signalling to the uterus to shed the endometrium, and you get a period. The pituitary gland reacts to the fall by increasing the level of FSH, and so a new cycle begins.

You may take the pattern of your menstrual cycle for granted, but it is very important from a biological point of view. The set pattern of hormonal messages between the pituitary gland and the ovaries ensures everything happens in the right order and at roughly the right time. For example, the egg will die if it arrives in the uterus before the lining – the endometrium – has been grown to support and nourish it. Your next period should only take place if you are not pregnant, otherwise you will lose the fertilised egg. Not surprisingly, the system can go wrong; ovulation or a period can be delayed by emotional upset, illness or poor diet, for example.

The way hormones control the menstrual cycle can be altered to prevent ovulation and pregnancy by taking the pill, which contains doses of oestrogen and progesterone. When you stop taking the pill for seven days, the hormone levels fall and you have a 'period'. Doctors call this a withdrawal bleed because your body has been 'tricked' into shedding the endometrium by withdrawing the hormones. They often say it is not a real period because you would not have it unless you stopped taking the tablets. It may be lighter and less painful than your natural period.

Understanding your anatomy and the menstrual cycle will help explain where endometriosis is found and how it is affected by hormonal messages (see Chapter 2) and, in turn, how artificial hormones can be used to treat it (see Chapter 3).

2
UNDERSTANDING ENDOMETRIOSIS

He showed me on a model where the endometriosis was and that it is blood shedding itself. How it was getting there – behind the womb, just outside – I do not know.

The ectopic occurrence of endometrial tissue or its diffuse implantation or infiltration in the myometrium.

Stedman's Medical Dictionary

Even when doctors do have time to explain, endometriosis is not easy to understand. Women often feel confused but are reluctant to ask 'dumb' questions. And resorting to a medical dictionary is not usually much help.

This chapter explains what endometriosis is, how it is diagnosed and why there can be problems and delays. It also looks at who gets endometriosis and how it might be caused.

WHAT IS ENDOMETRIOSIS?

The word endometriosis comes from endometrium, the lining of the uterus. If you have endometriosis this means that patches of tissue a bit like the endometrium have been found growing in parts of the body where they do not belong. But rest assured, endometriosis is *not* cancer. It is usually found on the perito-neum – the membrane lining the abdominal cavity – and on the surfaces of the organs in the pelvis. The illustration on page 11 will remind you how the organs fit neatly side by side in the pelvis with their surfaces touching each other, more or less covered by the peritoneum.

Endometriosis used to be described as clusters of bluish-black

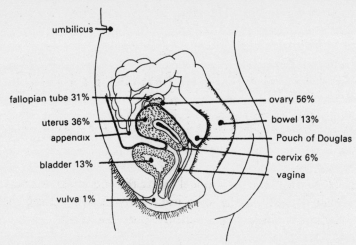

Where endometriosis can be found in the pelvis. (Percentage figures from the Endometriosis Society Survey. Rarer sites – umbilicus and appendix – not in survey.)

markings 'like powder burns' or old blood blisters. However, further research has shown that endometriosis can also appear as red, brown or white patches, clear bubble or flame-like blotches which apparently change over time into the more familiar bluish-black markings. Patches of endometriosis can be anything from microscopic to 2 cm across.

Endometriosis is most commonly found on the ovaries, but it can also be scattered on the uterus and its ligaments, the Fallopian tubes, the bowel or in the pouch of Douglas. Other sites such as the intestines, appendix, bladder, behind the navel, and on the lungs are far more rare. Occasionally endometriosis is found around the cervix, in the vagina or actually outside on the vaginal lips, and a few women have suffered from endometriosis in places such as the kidneys, pancreas or in more distant parts of the body like the arms, legs or head. An early record of endometriosis was made at Moorfields, the famous eye hospital. In fact, one review states that the only place endometriosis hasn't been noted is in the spleen!

Endometriosis can also appear in scars from surgery such as caesarean section or episiotomy and doctors acknowledge the endometrium can be accidently transplanted during surgery quite easily. In one small study in the early 1960s, doctors even deliberately implanted endometrium into the top of the vagina of 100 hysterectomy patients, so they continued to have cyclical bleeding and feel like 'real' women!

If endometriosis is diagnosed in any of the above sites you will it described in many gynaecology textbooks as 'external' endometriosis, because it occurs outside the uterus. 'Internal' endometriosis will be described as occurring inside the muscular wall of the uterus, and given the name adenomyosis. Researchers no longer talk in these terms because they believe adenomyosis is a different problem – most women with adenomyosis do not have endometriosis anywhere else and it is much less common. Your medical dictionary may be equally out-of-date on this (see, for example, the dictionary definition at the beginning of this chapter).

Although patches of endometriosis are outside the uterus, they can still be reached by hormones in the bloodstream. Chapter 1 discussed the hormonal changes that occur during the menstrual cycle and the diagram on pages 6–7 illustrates how patches of endometriosis respond to these changes. Like normal endometrium, endometriosis grows in response to the female hormone oestrogen and may bleed slightly when hormone levels fall at the end of the cycle and your period starts (although this is not proven).

Inflammation often develops around these patches, causing pain. The peritoneum is particularly sensitive to this irritation. Scar tissue then forms around the patches, but each cycle involves more endometriosis growth and bleeding. Endometriosis on the ovaries can develop into endometrioma or 'chocolate' cysts – clumps of old blood which are either the result of monthly bleeding or an increase in blood vessels around the damaged site. These cysts have been known to reach the size of oranges. However, finding a 'chocolate' cyst does not automatically mean there is endometriosis in the ovary; one study found up to 40 per cent of 'chocolate' cysts were caused in other ways.

Over time the constant build-up of scar tissue at different sites can lead to adhesions, best imagined as a kind of dense cling-film binding the organs together. Normally your organs slide gently against one another, but if you remember how neatly everything

☆ PAINFUL PERIODS
  TOTAL MENTION — 94%
  MILD — 6%
  MODERATE — 22%
  SEVERE — 66%
 PAINFUL OVULATION — 77%
 SWOLLEN ABDOMEN — 77%
 LOSS OF STALE BROWN BLOOD — 72%
 PRE MENSTRUAL TENSION — 67%
 DEPRESSION — 63%
 LOSS OF LARGE CLOTS DURING PERIOD — 62%
 PAIN AT ANY TIME — 57%
☆ PAINFUL SEX — 55%
 HEAVY BLEEDING — 48%
☆ PAINFUL DEFAECATION — 48%
 CONSTIPATION — 45%
 NAUSEA — 42%
 BACK PAIN
  DURING PERIODS — 37%
  MOST OF THE TIME — 42%
☆ INFERTILITY — 41%
 DIZZINESS — 33%
 IRREGULAR PERIODS — 34%
 DIARRHOEA — 27%
☆ PAINFUL URINATION — 26%
 INSOMNIA — 21%
  DUE TO PAIN — 32%
 PSYCHOLOGICAL SYMPTOMS — 15%
 OTHER — 13%

☆ TEXTBOOK SYMPTOMS

Symptoms described by over 700 sufferers in the Endometriosis Society Survey.

fits in the pelvis you can see how easily the ovaries might stick to the uterus or how the uterus might stick to the bowel, perhaps with one or both ovaries caught in between. Inflammation around endometriosis and subsequent adhesions can cause a range of problems.

SYMPTOMS

The symptoms emphasised in medical textbooks are one or more of the following:

- Infertility
- Painful periods (dysmenorrhoea)
- Painful sexual intercourse (dyspareunia)
- Painful bowel movements or urination

You might like to compare this with the table which illustrates what more than 700 sufferers said were symptoms of their endometriosis in their opinion. It is striking how much pain many women suffer, whether it is severe painful periods (66 per cent), painful ovulation (77 per cent), painful sex (55 per cent), painful urination (26 per cent) or painful bowel movements (48 per cent). There is thus no doubt that endometriosis can be an extremely painful disease in many cases. Yet some sufferers do not have any symptoms at all. They may not even realise they have got endometriosis until it is discovered by accident when surgery is performed for a completely different reason – 8 per cent of women in the Endometriosis Society survery said their endometriosis was found during another operation and other studies have shown endometriosis in up to 22 per cent of women without symptoms undergoing sterilisation.

It was thought the discrepancy between the amount of endometriosis and painful symptoms could be explained by looking at where patches were found rather than their size. Although there is some relationship, further detailed work on the structure of endometriosis suggests that this isn't the whole story. When researchers looked at how deep the endometriosis went they discovered that the deeper the sites, the more likely a woman was to have painful symptoms. Deep lesions (more than 5 mm) appear to be an older more active stage of endometriosis and sometimes contain nerve fibres, suggesting a reason for the link with painful symptoms. Furthermore, they were more likely to be found around the pouch of Douglas or uterosacral ligaments where they may cause pain during sexual intercourse or bowel movements.

Many symptoms of endometriosis are worse just before or during a period and many doctors will look for this cyclical pattern when making a diagnosis. For example, your bowel movements or urination may become painful regularly around this time, and in severe cases blood may appear in your stools or urine. Recent studies found deeply infiltrating patches of endometriosis often change in phase with the normal endometrium, suggesting an explanation for cyclical painful symptoms. (However, research has also suggested that endometriosis can change in an unpredictable way and it may be unhelpful to assume it is like normal endometrium.) The regular build-up of inflammation and adhesions may lead to acute pain at any time or persistent pain throughout the month, and in time, adhesions can prove to be a more painful problem than the endometriosis itself.

Pain is one of the most distressing aspects of the disease, capable of eroding your way of life, and affecting your confidence in yourself and others.

I *hate* pain, it invades me.

I was convinced that the continued pain meant I would never recover and that I had not been told the truth.

On days free from pain or discomfort I feel great and can cope with any situation. When I do not feel well even answering the telephone is traumatic. I feel exhausted and my work is suffering.

Low energy level, lethargy and tiredness because of constant pain – day and night. Erratic mood changes. This general 'unreasonableness' was a major cause of conflict with my husband, also lack of interest in sex.

I know (in my case) my chances of pregnancy are small, but they would be much better if I could only get rid of the pain for a little while. I could then forget my non-pregnant state, relax more and give myself a better chance of conceiving.

It is clear from sufferers' comments that pain produces a lot of problems and these often combine to make them feel tired miserable and out of control – 63 per cent in the survey said depression was a symptom of their endometriosis, 32 per cent complained of insomnia due to pain and 15 per cent mentioned various psychological problems. Most doctors would argue that tiredness and depression are not symptoms of endometriosis, but women count these feelings because they are describing what the whole experience of endometriosis can be like. For them, this includes problems caused directly by endometriosis, such as pain, and those it may cause indirectly, such as tiredness and depression. These feelings and ways in which pain and exhaustion can be managed are discussed in more detail in Chapters 8 and 9.

Another probable reason for the high level of depression reported in the survey is that 41 per cent had experienced infertility. Similar figures are given in other research. The association between endometriosis and infertility, and how women experience this problem, are explored in Chapter 6.

DIAGNOSIS

At present there is no quick simple test for endometriosis. Your doctor can check the position of the uterus and find certain signs that suggest endometriosis and exclude other possibilities during a pelvic examination.

Quite a lot of women have a retroverted uterus (see page 4) but this position is more common among endometriosis sufferers, where the uterus may be difficult to move because it is stuck to the bowel with adhesions. Your doctor your also be able to feel suspicious lumps, or that the ovaries are enlarged. Painful sexual intercourse is quite often associated with tender nodules in the pouch of Douglas or uterosacral ligaments, so your doctor may try and reproduce this pain by prodding and stretching this area (be warned!). Sometimes thickenings in the ligaments due to patches of endometriosis can be felt if the vagina and rectum are both examined at the same time.

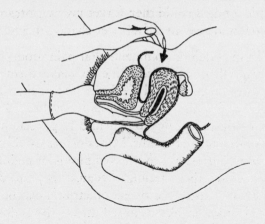

Feeling the position of the uterus.

However, the usual way to diagnose endometriosis is to look for it. If you think back to where endometriosis is usually found (see page 11), you will realise that growths scattered around the pelvis cannot be seen by looking up the vagina – they can only be seen by looking inside the abdomen (except in rare cases where they occur beyond the pelvis). In the past this involved major abdominal surgery, but nowadays, a minor operation known as a laparoscopy is done instead.

Laparoscopy

A laparoscopy is usually a very quick operation under general anaesthetic, lasting 10–20 minutes. Carbon dioxide gas is pumped into the abdomen (they do let it out again) before an incision is made near the navel to insert the laparoscope, which lights up and magnifies the pelvic organs where endometriosis is usually found. Sometimes a second incision is made lower down and another instrument is used to move the organs slightly to look around and behind them. You will be in hospital for one or two days and may take a week or so to get back to normal after the operation. Your abdomen will feel tender and swollen at first, and there will be the usual after-effects of a general anaesthetic, e.g. possible nausea, tiredness, weakness. Some women complain of shoulder pains after a laparoscopy; this is because any carbon dioxide gas left behind will collect under the diaphragm (the sheet of muscle between the abdomen and the chest) and cause referred pain (pain felt in a different part of the body) in your shoulders.

Some assessment of the severity of the endometriosis will be made at laparoscopy. Medical texts outline ways of judging stages of endometriosis based on the number of sites and extent of adhesions (see below). However this does not necessarily relate to symptoms; you may be diagnosed as having mild endometriosis, with a few patches in the pouch of Douglas or on the uterine ligaments, and yet be in agony. Equally, it doesn't reflect how far endometriosis may have infiltrated into the tissue. Detailed work has shown a small patch may have a quite extensive system 'underground'. Researchers are trying to develop a more relevant classification system to take account of these points.

Laparoscopy is now routinely performed to check the diagnosis of several gynaecological problems. The laparoscope is also used in infertility investigations and sterilisations. It is certainly a great improvement on major surgery of the past, but it is not an entirely foolproof method of diagnosing endometriosis. Endometriosis may be missed during the operation for various reasons. For a start, researchers have demonstrated that endometriosis can be microscopic – too small to see with a laparoscope. They may not recognise some of the more unusual appearances of endometriosis as, for example, colourless blisters (see page 11). One review suggests that microscopic or unrecognised endometriosis is missed by surgeons in up to 6 per cent of cases. Even if endometriosis is potentially visible, it may be tucked away where it is difficult to see with the laparoscope, especially if adjacent organs are stuck together with adhesions. Adhesions in the absence of visible endometriosis could indicate other problems such as pelvic inflammatory disease (PID).

Some doctors have suggested that a laparoscopy for suspected endometriosis should be done just before a period, when the disease may be most active and easier to see. Although a few hospital wards try to ensure a woman is booked in late in her cycle, most do not make this special arrangement because of the lack of agreement on its value and the considerable organisation involved.

A few gynaecologists are now advising a second look for

women who have a negative laparoscopy (i.e. nothing was found) but who continue to suffer debilitating symptoms. One doctor reports finding the worst case of endometriosis he had ever seen at a second-look laparoscopy, when the first laparoscopy just nine months earlier showed a clear pelvis. This case is dramatic enough to prove the point, but in the absence of more information about how long endometriosis takes to become visible it is difficult for doctors to recommend when the second look should take place. Hospitals wishing to employ this strategy also have to cope with limited resources for re-laparoscopy and GPs' difficulty in making a second gynaecological diagnosis when laparoscopy has revealed nothing.

In some countries, particularly the United States, diagnosis is only confirmed if a biopsy (a small sample of tissue) shows

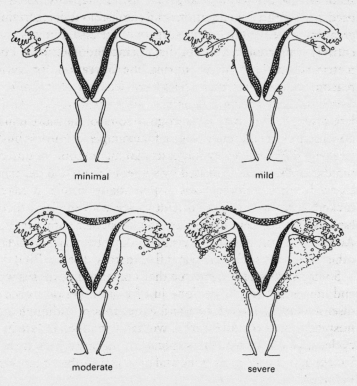

minimal   mild

moderate   severe

Visible degrees of endometriosis.

endometriosis cells under the microscope. This procedure avoids mistaking other bleeding and blemishes seen during laparoscopy that are not due to endometriosis. However, a problem remains: Where do you take the biopsy from if you cannot see any endometriosis during laparoscopy? It is possible to take it from the wrong place and still miss the endometriosis. On the other hand, biopsies of normal-looking peritoneum have found endometriosis in an unexpected number of cases so microscopic endometriosis may be very common. It has been argued that it could be so common as to occur in most women some of the time, without causing significant problems. If it does occur 'normally' in this way, it could be that the more you look for it, then the more you'll find it. Then the questions are whether such patches are likely to progress and cause problems or not and if they should be treated just because they are there. When is endometriosis without symptoms just endometrium in the wrong place and when is it a disease? Researchers are still arguing.

Rare cases where women have endometriosis beyond the pelvis will also be missed at laparoscopy. These cases can be very difficult to diagnose unless *someone* notices the pattern of bleeding at these sites:

I had an ultrasound scan which revealed a large piece of tissue which was bleeding at the time (during my period). After a liver scan and X-ray which did not reveal a malignant lump, doctors decided that it could be endometriosis as it only seemed to bleed during my period causing severe pain and discomfort.

After coughing blood the chest X-ray showed a shadow on the lung – 10 days later it had disappeared. This continued for about 4 months and the chest physician was mystified as all other diagnoses had been ruled out. When I said to him how strange I thought it was that it occurred during the first few days of menstruation, bells started to ring and a gynaecologist was consulted. When the pattern had established itself over the next few months endometriosis was diagnosed.

An accurated diagnosis of endometriosis is important partly because treatment is different from that for other gynaecological or bowel problems with which it may be confused, but also because it is generally thought that endometriosis builds up inflammation and scar tissue every month if left untreated. However, few studies suggest that endometriosis does not always get worse. It appears that only one third of women with endometriosis may have progressive disease. In the other two thirds, it may remain the same or spontaneously heal. Since doctors cannot predict yet which endometriosis sufferers are likely to improve or worsen, they still have to treat everyone. These findings also make it difficult to judge whether any improvements after treatment are due to the treatment itself or the disease improving of its own accord.

Future diagnostic tests

Researchers have been looking for ways to diagnose endometriosis without surgery, and one way is to look at the production of antigens and antibodies. The body's immune system reacts to 'foreign' chemicals (known as antigens) and invading infections by producing antibodies – chemicals of its own that clump around and try to neutralise or knock out the 'foreign' antigen or infection.

A blood test for endometriosis was suggested after high levels of an antigen, CA-125, were found circulating in the blood of some women with severe endometriosis. Further work showed that a CA-125 blood test could detect some severe cases, but other women had normal CA-125 blood levels in spite of having extensive endometriosis, and the test was even more unreliable in women with mild disease. However, further work showed that while this technique was good at finding problems if they were there, it wasn't good enough at telling the difference between endometriosis and other problems such as pelvic adhesions or pelvic inflammatory disease.

Work was also done on CA-125 combined with a diagnostic technique called immunoscintigraphy. The idea is to give an injection of antibodies against CA-125 marked with a tiny, safe amount of radioactivity. The antibodies become concentrated in areas of endometriosis which can then be seen on pictures taken with a special machine that detects areas of radioactivity. This test does not depend on the levels of the CA-125 antigen circulating in the bloodstream, as the radioactive-labelled antibodies produced by the body go to the sites where the CA-125 is produced.

It looks like some of these techniques might prove useful in monitoring endometriosis, but not in diagnosing it in the first place.

Getting a referral

Laparoscopy is not a simple test health centres can use to screen women, so it remains for your GP to arrive at a provisional diagnosis and refer you to a specialist for further investigation. To reach this stage both you and your GP have to agree that you have got a problem which needs specialist attention. You have got to respond to your symptoms by making initial or repeated visits; your GP must decide what your problem is likely to be and whether to treat you, refer you or ask you to come back if the problem persists. All sorts of delay can occur before you get a referral.

The Endometriosis Society survey tried to find out which symptoms prompted endometriosis sufferers to visit their GPs in the beginning. Replies suggest that infertility and severe period pains prompted sufferers to make the first visit more often than embarrassing symptoms such as painful sex or painful defaecation. For example, 66 per cent of women in the survey suffered from very painful periods and just under half said this is what prompted them to visit their doctor. However 55 per cent suffered from painful sex, but only one in five of these women said this pain prompted them to seek medical advice.

Many sufferers also describe how they delayed going to their doctors because they thought their symptoms were a 'normal' part of being a woman.

I just kept putting it down to other things, premenstrual tension, problems with relationships, the pressures of bringing up two children.

Making love really hurt deep down in certain positions. I just

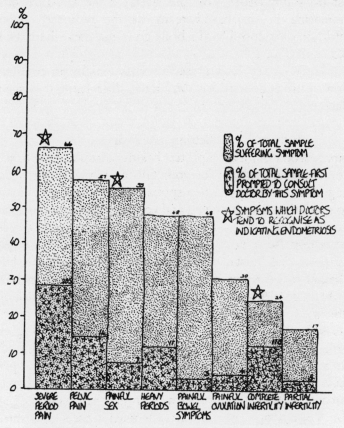

RESULTS FROM ENDOMETRIOSIS SOCIETY SURVEY – 726 WOMEN

Symptoms first prompting women to visit their GP.

thought, well, either he was too long or I was too short. How was I supposed to know? A friend said I ought to mention the pain to my doctor.

Some anticipated that their doctors would agree.

I feel doctors generally think pain is part of periods and we should put up with it – I thought this too, but it can mean that anyone with endometriosis does not seek help until it is really bad. What is bad pain? I always thought if I stand it then it must be bearable – maybe it would have been better if I'd fainted.

It can be very difficult to communicate your symptoms. Saying you cannot conceive is straightforward, but how do you convey just how much pain you are experiencing or how serious you feel things are.

My own doctor told me period pains were something women had to put up with, which infuriated me because I had explained that the pains I was having were far more than my ordinary period pains. I had not been able to conceive for two years and I was at the end of my tether with such dreadful pains.

You cannot produce proof of how you feel and therefore begin to wonder if you are exaggerating your symptoms when all the time you know you are being honest with yourself.

You may also be worried about your GP's response to 'feminine' complaints. The popular image of the neurotic female patient is all too familiar to endometriosis sufferers who feel their doctors did not take them seriously in the beginning. It is a recurring theme in stories of misdiagnosis:

Spastic colon, cystitis, neuroses.

Psychological – lack of commitment in my life!

Appendicitis, bowel spasms, chronic back pain, lack of sex causing congestion in the pelvis, retroverted uterus, over-active thyroid, neurosis.

He was convinced I had a kidney disorder. Everything else was in my mind. All he wanted to do was prescribe Valium.

Year 1: Stress, neurosis, psychosomatic.
Year 2: Menstrual troubles, 'will settle down', appendicitis?

Year 3: Ovarian cyst diagnosed by GP, consultant says I'm 100 per cent OK and tries to refer me to someone to 'talk about it'.
Year 4: Endometriosis.

'Suffering from acute depression' – that was what the doctor said. Seven hours later I was rushed into hospital and had an emergency operation in which they removed one ovary, one tube and appendix. Since then I found out they found endometriosis.

Many sufferers report that their doctors diagnosed their complaints as psychosomatic. The term 'psychosomatic' is often misused by doctors and the general public alike. Your doctor may mean there is nothing physically wrong with you and that it is all in your head (which is hysteria) or that you are exaggerating minor symptoms (hypochondriasis). Psychosomatic means your emotions (psyche) have produced a physiological effect on your body (soma). Psychological factors may contribute to the development of endometriosis (see Chapter 8), but this should not prevent recognition of a real physical disease requiring treatment. Equally, even if a woman is suffering from severe mental illness, she may still have endometriosis. Understanding is not helped by gynaecology textbooks which make statements such as 'girls' experience period pains because 'their outlook on sex, health and menstruation is faulty'.

Few women would deny that symptoms such as severe period pains or painful sexual activity are associated with emotional upset. However, they see this as the natural result of such pain, not the cause.

I felt a lack of knowledge and terror [about the pain] – which leads to neurosis which doctors then diagnose.

Several times over the last few years I have been told my problem is psychosomatic – a couple of years before endometriosis was diagnosed the doctor said the answer was to get married and have a baby! I felt so ill I burst into tears – which seemed to confirm the diagnosis!

One of the problems is obviously doctors' attitudes towards women complaining of this sort of pain – they always seem to think 'She is neurotic, therefore she says she is in pain.' They never think 'She is anxious because she *is* in pain.'

The apparent contradiction between emotions and stress contributing to a disease on the one hand, and being a natural reaction to being ill on the other, is best understood as part of a vicious circle. For example, you probably will be anxious because you are in pain; equally your pain may also get worse as you become more anxious. These ideas are explored further in Chapters 8 and 9.

Even if you are able to communicate your symptoms and your GP keeps an open mind and is up to date, he or she may not refer you on your first visit. Endometriosis can be very hard to diagnose because individual symptoms vary so much and could indicate other gynaecological problems (such as pelvic inflammatory disease) or be mistaken for a range of bowel and bladder complaints (e.g. cystitis, spastic colon and irritable bowel syndrome). In addition, GPs are not experienced gynecologists and do not have the benefit of a laparoscope, so short of referring every woman with painful periods to a specialist, many GPs wait and see if problems get worse and patients come back. This is illustrated in the Endometriosis Society survey, which showed that 41 per cent were only referred to a gynaecologist after repeated visits to their GP. Thirty-three per cent were referred straightaway, and this was more likely if the symptoms reported included infertility. The fact that 11 per cent were treated by their GPs for something else and 6 per cent were first referred to specialists other than gynaecologists may reflect lack of awareness of endometriosis, lack of up-to-date information and technical difficulty in making the diagnosis.

While 'wait and see' may be a reasonable strategy from your GP's point of view, it is tough on you if you are the one whose painful periods *are* due to a gynaecological problem such as endometriosis. You cannot do much about your GP's workload or medical education, but there are several things you can do if you feel you are not getting medical attention for the symptoms described earlier. The first thing is to go back to your GP; the survey shows that just because your GP did not refer you the first time, this does not mean he or she would not refer you next time. However this may be easier said than done when you have had to screw up your courage once already!

Fear and reluctance to discuss embarrassing symptoms are understandable but can also be counterproductive. In the absence of infertility, painful sex is one of the signs most likely to lead GPs to consider the possibility of endometriosis. Research has also shown that painful sex is the symptom most likely to predict a subsequent finding of endometriosis. Charting your menstrual cycle can provide useful information for you and your doctor since it will help you notice any changes. A pain scale (see Chapter 9) can help you record your pain. If possible, visit your GP when you actually have symptoms so he or she will be able to get a better idea of the problem. If you think you have got endometriosis, try suggesting it.

If you are concerned about your doctor's response the try writing down what you want to say. Plan to ask for what you feel you need (e.g. referral to a gynaecologist, pain relief, etc.). At least your GP may then give reasons if he or she does not agree, rather than simply not realising your concerns. Talk it over with a friend or partner beforehand to check you have thought it through. It may also help to take someone with you for moral support. If you have difficulty understanding what your GP says, ask him or her to repeat or clarify it. Make notes if it helps. If you do not think your GP has understood what you have said then check, or try repeating it a different way. If you do not agree with your GP's comments then do question them (yes, this can be hard). Doctors are human so being pleasant to them usually produces a better response (of course, this applies equally to patients!). Although it is easier to say nothing and perhaps accept tablets which you know you will not take, you will end up worrying and visiting your GP all over again. If you feel rushed into discussing things when you feel uncomfortable or embarrassed ('I would have liked doctors to talk to my face, not my bottom'), then ask for a minute until you are ready.

If all this seems impossible, then it may help to get some practice and support in being assertive. The most articulate woman who can stand up and talk to large audiences, run a playgroup or even take defective shoes back to a shop may come out of the surgery furious with herself for not saying what she meant to. Some people can only wind themselves up to say what they really want to if they get very angry or very upset, but they usually feel awful afterwards and this approach tends to be counterproductive. Learning to be assertive can be extremely helpful and make you feel much more confident and positive (see the recommended list on page 159; assertiveness training courses may be available locally).

YOU AND THE NHS

What you can expect as a right

- The services of a GP. You do not have to give reasons for changing doctors, but the new doctor is not obliged to take you. Contact your Family Health Services Authority (FHSA).
- To receive appropriate medical services, as judged by what other doctors would have done in the same situation, e.g. home visits.
- To be informed about substantial risks of treatment. Your consultant has wide discretion about what constitutes adequate information; ask about any treatment which is suggested.
- To have an abortion, sterilisation or any other operation without your husband's consent.
- To apply to see your medical records and to have them to be kept confidential from people not concerned with your treatment.

What you cannot expect as a right

- A home visit, if your doctor does not agree your circumstances require it in medical terms.
- A second opinion, although it is normally recognised as being an 'appropriate medical service'.

What you do not have to agree to

- Any particular medical examination or treatment. Treatment without your consent is assault, except in certain emergencies. Consent forms for operations are currently being

improved. Discuss this with your doctor if you are worried. You do not have to take part in medical research.
- Having medical students present when you are examined. You have a right to be informed about this, and to be invited to give your consent. Further details are given in copies of *The Patient's Charter* available from libraries, etc. You can also write to your Patient's Charter Officer at your local FHSA; contact your local Community Health Council or ring The National Health Information Line on freephone 0800 665544.

You may decide to change your GP. You can try seeing one of the other doctors in the practice or a locum – a doctor who takes over when your doctor's away. You do not need a letter from your GP to attend a family planning clinic, cervical cytology clinic or venereal ('special') clinic, so you could try talking to doctors there – they cannot usually refer you to a gynaecologist without your GP's consent, but a letter could carry some weight. If you do want to change your GP follow the directions on your medical card or discuss the problem with your local Family Health Services Authority (FHSA). They will have a list of local GPs and their special interests and be able to advise you (in some places, the FHSA may have become part of a purchasing authority and be known by a variety of names, e.g. Xshire Health or Xshire Health Commission). Your local Community Health Council or CHC (look in the Yellow Pages under 'Community') is another source of help. The local CHC is the patients' voice in the area and is there to help you with problems and complaints.

WHO GETS ENDOMETRIOSIS?

Although most people have never heard of it, endometriosis is a common disease estimated to affect between 1–15 per cent of women. It is the second most common gynaecological disorder after fibroids, and is diagnosed in about 25 per cent of gynaecological operations.

Researchers are now beginning to look at who gets endometriosis, if it is more common in certain groups, and whether there

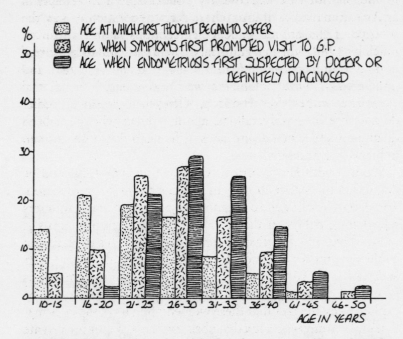

Age of sufferers when they felt they began to suffer, when they first visited their GP, and when they were finally diagnosed. (An Endometriosis Society Survey of 726 women.)

are risk factors which increase the chances of the disease developing. This kind of information could alert a doctor when making a diagnosis, and understanding risk factors can make prevention easier. Equally, inaccurate information can hinder diagnosis.

Endometriosis is associated with menstruation, so it does not occur before puberty. However, many doctors are not up-to-date with reports that endometriosis can occur in women after the menopause, whether it be natural or surgical, e.g. if a woman is on hormone replacement therapy (HRT) or if fragments of ovarian tissue remain after surgery. Although both these occurences are rare, they can be severe and women who have had such an experience were not helped by their doctors' lack of awareness (see Chapter 4).

Endometriosis has often been characterised as a disease most commonly suffered by white middle-class middle-aged women in spite of evidence to the contrary. For example, a 1954 paper in an American medical journal characterised endometriosis as 'the scourge of the private patient'. Perceptions hadn't advanced much by 1980, when an editorial in the *British Medical Journal* quoted endometriosis sufferers as predominantly white and middle-class. Such statements were often based on clinical experience rather than research, but even in research studies doctors are inevitably talking about women who have been diagnosed and when a disease is difficult to diagnose this can influence the findings.

Women with endometriosis can have no symptoms and be diagnosed by chance during an appendectomy or sterilisation. The disease is difficult to diagnose anyway, and many sufferers report long delays in diagnosis. So perhaps endometriosis is more commonly *diagnosed* in certain groups. This explanation could account for some of the past statements about who gets endometriosis. For example, the suggestion that endometriosis is more common amongst higher social classes could be explained by the fact that these women often have the information and resources to get a diagnosis, perhaps by seeking private consultations more often. In general, white women also have greater access to resources and so may also be diagnosed more often than non-white women. Recent research papers show that doctors have become more aware of these issues and it is now argued that endometriosis appears to affect different races and social classes equally when confounding factors are taken into account. However, your doctor may not be up-to-date.

The hospital doctor did say it was rare in Afro-Carribean women.

Endometriosis was also seen as a disease of middle-aged women (perhaps reflecting how long it took to get diagnosed!). There is mounting evidence that the risk of developing endometriosis increases with the number of menstrual cycles a woman experiences over time, explaining why it is more commonly diagnosed as women become older, but there are also numerous papers which agree that endometriosis in young women is not rare. For example, one research paper notes that endometriosis was found in 47–65 per cent of teenagers complaining of persistent pelvic pain or painful sex. Another review reports the average age of diagnosis as 25 to 29 years, although the authors suggest better methods of diagnosing microscopic or unusual, early forms of endometriosis might bring this average down (although see the debate about whether endometriosis is a disease in early cases without symptoms on page 20).

Another unhelpful notion in early medical and magazine articles was endometriosis being 'the career woman's disease'. There is no evidence that endometriosis is more common amongst women who have delayed child-bearing in favour of their job rather than for other reasons, and all sorts of factors would need to be taken into account before supporting such a view. For example, endometriosis is associated with infertility so a pattern of late pregnancies amongst such a group could be explained by reduced fertility rather than choice of occupation. Indeed, such women could have pursued their occupation on this basis.

> I find the idea that I'm a 'career woman' and therefore somehow unmotherly very hurtful when I would have loved to have had children.

A recent American study actually set out 'to examine the belief that women with endometriosis have "voluntarily" delayed childbirth' and found no significant difference between women with endometriosis and two groups of other women in factors such as birth control, sexual activity, decisions with regard to pregnancy, age at first pregnancy, etc. As the researchers concluded, the notion of endometriosis patients as career women is an unsupported simplistic assumption.

Arguments about who gets endometriosis will continue for as long as it is impractical to screen all women for endometriosis. In the meantime, statements about the 'typical sufferer' need to be treated with caution.

Endometriosis in families

Research suggests that about 7 per cent of women with endometriosis have a close relative who also suffers. A similar proportion (8 per cent) of the 726 women in the Endometriosis

Society survey reported endometriosis in their families. These figures do not necessarily mean that endometriosis is inherited; they might just mean it is so common that more than one person in a family will develop it. However, there is some work which argues that endometriosis is an inherited disease and this is now an active area of international research. No one is sure why it only happens in some families and not others, but when it does, it can bring its own special problems and worries.

In June my younger unmarried sister started to complain of stabbing pains which were quite severe in her side. On hearing about me the consultant said she could have endometriosis. She went in for a laparoscopy and was found to have slight endometriosis. She has been put on danazol for 4–6 months. I have been able to help her, as no one was for me, by explaining things, reassuring, etc. My Mum is now blaming herself, which I keep telling her is silly. She is convinced that she did something wrong whilst she was bringing us up. I think she is the most upset of the three of us – one daughter having endometriosis was bad enough, but two!

When my endometriosis was discovered two years ago, my mother told me that she had suffered the same thing. She ended up having a hysterectomy where her consultant described the inside of her as if someone had taken a tube of glue and stuck everything together [adhesions]. I am the eldest of three girls but fortunately they have escaped it. I am hoping some research will be done on this as I have a beautiful young daughter (aged five) and would hate to think she will suffer in years to come.

One of the striking features of other stories is how much endometriosis can vary between sisters, or even between identical twins.

It is interesting to compare our symptoms – I had it very badly and no pain, my sister had lots of pain and only slightly.

I have an identical twin sister who has just been diagnosed, following painful periods for the last six months or so. I find it interesting that she has only recently developed the symptoms whereas my own endometriosis has been evident for nearly ten years now (we are both 29).

Of course, if members of families have similar symptoms, that can have disadvantages.

I finally screwed up courage to ask my mother about the deep sharp pains I felt during sex. She told me she'd had them for years and you could avoid them by only using certain positions. Later a medical friend said I should go and see a doctor. I told my Mum she should too. We both ended up having laparoscopies and endometriosis was diagnosed. I was 22, she was 47. So far my two younger sisters are fine.

WHAT CAUSES IT?

Medical theories

No one really knows why endometriosis occurs. There are plenty of theories which are difficult or impossible to test. The most popular one suggests the disease results from 'retrograde menstruation', when muscle spasms during a period force menstrual blood backwards up the Fallopian tubes and into the pelvic cavity, where it can form endometriosis. To understand how this can happen, it is important to realise that each Fallopian tube has a feathery end which opens out next to the ovary (see Chapter 1). There is a small gap between the ovary and the tube's entrance. Normally, when an egg is released it is guided across the gap and into the tube by the feathery 'fingers', and then passes on its way to the uterus. If menstrual blood is squeezed backwards up either Fallopian tube, it will leak into this gap between the 'fingers' and the ovary and then out around the organs.

The retrograde menstruation theory may explain why endometriosis is most commonly found on the ovaries, because this is the first place the stray menstrual blood is likely to land.

However, research suggests that retrograde menstruation is common amongst all women, not just endometriosis sufferers. The theory does not explain why endometriosis occurs in the lungs and other distant places.

Another theory suggests that endometrial tissue is carried from the womb to other parts of the body via the lymph (fluid in the tissues) or blood, but again this does not account for why the condition only develops in certain women. Yet another idea, the metaplasia theory, states that cells in the body are converted to endometrial cells by recurring infection, hormone imbalance, or polluting chemicals (e.g. dioxin).

Endometriosis has been reported in one or two men treated with female hormones for various cancers, e.g. cancer of the prostate gland. This observation tends to argue against the retrograde menstruation theory for obvious reasons and supports the metaplasia theory since cells must have changed into endometrial cells as a result of the high levels of the female hormones administered.

It has also been proposed that remnants of a woman's prenatal (before birth) tissue develop into endometriosis. At a very early stage in life, when a baby girl is growing in her mother's womb, certain cells are programmed to change into the female organs. It is thought that some of these cells can end up in the wrong place. When the girl begins to menstruate these areas respond to her hormones just like the normal endometrium because they came from the same foetal tissue.

There has been considerable interest in the more recent idea that women with endometriosis have an immune deficiency, i.e. the body's immune system is in some way defective. A weak immune system may allow endometriosis to develop as a result of retrograde menstruation or endometrial cells circulating in the lymphatic (tissue fluid) system, explaining why some women have the disease and not others. Some women with endometriosis have also been found to have unexpectedly high levels of antibodies which attack cells of some of their own organs, e.g. auto-antibodies to the thyroid. Immunology is a very complicated area of study so it will be sometime before researchers can decide whether endometriosis is a fact an auto-immune disease and explain how it occurs.

Your theories

'Why me?' is a natural question when one is faced with a chronic, often painful, disease such as endometriosis. Most sufferers have some feeling about what caused their endometriosis, even if they just put it down to fate. In the Endometriosis Society survey, family history, stress (in general, a specific trauma or due to work), previous contraceptives, doctors' neglect, God's will and fate were most often ticked as possible influences on the development of endometriosis.

Women who replied to the survey were concerned about possible effects of the pill and IUD (the coil). There is no evidence that the pill stimulates the development of endometriosis; in fact researchers have argued that it could have a protective effect. The IUD often causes heavy, painful periods and some sufferers feel this led to their endometriosis. However many women get period problems with the IUD without developing endometriosis so, in the absence of research, it seems unlikely that the IUD causes endometriosis on its own.

Some women feel their endometriosis might have been caused by using tampons – a third of the 726 women replying to the survey said they had given up using tampons because of discomfort. It has been suggested that tampon use might increase the amount of retrograde menstruation and hence the chances of developing endometriosis. However, a study of tampon use amongst 470 members of the American Endometriosis Association found no evidence that tampon use was related to endometriosis.

3
DRUG TREATMENTS

My GP's comment was that I'll be better when I reach the menopause. With only 27 years to go, I can't wait!

Endometriosis can be treated in the short-term, but in the longer term it is likely to recur and there is no guaranteed cure, although it is rare for it to continue beyond the menopause. The fact that endometriosis does not grow and bleed if there is no menstruation means that drugs which stop menstruation can be used to treat it. This chapter looks at the drugs your gynaecologist may prescribe. What is recommended will depend on your age, your desire to have children (or more), where your endometriosis is and the problems it is causing. It will also depend on your consultant's views on endometriosis and its treatment, and his/her familiarity with current research. In some cases, for example, if you have mild infertility and are keen to get pregnant, no treatment may be prescribed at all (see chapter 6).

It is worth noting that you and your doctors may have to experiment a little to find the right drug treatment for you. Individual sufferers can vary in their response to different drug treatments and research suggests this may be explained by variations in the type of receptors present in endometriosis. Receptors are perhaps best imagined as being like locks for keys, in this case hormone molecules. Another key may fit but not open the lock. Drugs often work by occupying a lock instead of the correct hormone molecule; if enough receptors are occupied but not unlocked the menstrual cycle will be disrupted. Similarly, if enough receptors on the endometriosis are occupied, its growth will be disrupted. The idea is that one drug may be better at 'fitting' the receptors on your endometriosis and therefore be more successful at relieving your symptoms.

Treatment is usually prescribed for six to nine months,

although some researchers are recommending this be reduced to three months because of evidence that if a drug is going to be effective it will have affected endometriosis cells after two months and reduced symptoms after three. This work also suggests that if changes in cell structure haven't occurred by this time, they aren't going to occur with continued use of the drug and so a different drug treatment should be tried. Your doctor(s) may not be aware of (or perhaps agree with) this research but it is worth going back to your GP if you feel the treatment isn't working or is causing other problems, particularly after two to three months when you've given it a fair chance.

DANAZOL

Danazol (marketed as Danol) was first described in 1971 and is the most common drug treatment for endometriosis; 75 per cent of sufferers in the Endometriosis Society survey had taken it. Danazol tricks the body into a fake or 'pseudo-menopause', although it is uncertain exactly how the drug works. However, the result is very low levels of the hormone oestrogen.

If you are given danazol your periods will probably stop, although this depends on the dose, which may be anything from 200–800 mg per day. If your dose is too low you may get breakthrough bleeding as your body tries to have a period; research shows that for the drug to be most effective the dose should be high enough to stop menstruation completely (amenorrhoea). One or two women have reported taking does as high as 1,200 mg per day; this is very high and if you are taking as much as this you should check with your doctor that it is really necessary. If you get any problems, discuss them with your doctor. There is no harm in you both adjusting the dose to find the right one for you – or in trying a different drug altogether.

You will usually be asked to start danazol after a period, to make sure that you are not pregnant – taking danazol during pregnancy can lead to a baby girl developing male characteristics. Danazol is only an effective contraceptive if taken at daily doses of 400 mg and above, so if you are taking less than 400 mg daily you should use a barrier contraceptive such as the condom or cap (although these methods are recommended for safer sex with regard to HIV irrespective of the need for contraception). Danazol is not recommended if you are epileptic, suffer from migraine, diabetes mellitus or heart, liver or kidney problems, and it should not be prescribed if you are breastfeeding.

Side effects

Danazol has a reputation for side effects and research suggests that 85 per cent of women are affected. Of the side effects reported in the Endometriosis Society survey, weight gain was the most common. Some side effects are related to the 'pseudo-menopause' danazol produces, e.g. hot flushes, dry vagina. Others, such as increased hair (hirsutism), acne and voice changes, occur because the drug is similar to the male hormone testosterone (but, you will be glad to hear, only one-tenth as strong). You will not necessarily get all these side effects or have them badly, and sometimes the number of side effects and their severity can be reduced by taking a lower dose.

Danazol arouses strong feelings amongst endometriosis sufferers. The side effects can be very depressing, but the relief from symptoms can make it all worthwhile. As with many other aspects of endometriosis, women tend to have different reactions and different needs.

I suffered shrinking breasts while taking it, but I still feel the benefits of being pain-free far outweigh the disadvantages.

The side effects of danazol were tolerable. I am thin anyway, so I didn't mind the weight gain, although my face looked puffy. I also had hot flushes, but these were OK. I found remembering to take the tablets worse than the side effects.

Some sufferers have found that vitamin B6 and/or evening primrose oil (see Chapter 5) help counteract feelings of depression and lethargy when on danazol. Others comment that dolomite (magnesium/calcium) helps with muscle cramps.

I would like to give some encouragement to people taking danazol. I have been taking 200 mg per day. I have offset feelings of depression and lethargy to a certain extent with

vitamin B6 and have managed to keep my weight steady after
an initial half-stone gain. I'm generally feeling better and
more energetic and able to cope with life. The added bonus is
no periods – even on this low dose. I have found that
modifying my diet to eat more fruit/veg and natural yoghurts
has also been beneficial – more fibre, fewer bowel problems
and fewer spots.

Most side effects usually disappear when treatment ends, but it is
generally accepted that singers should not take danazol because
the voice changes that occasionally occur are not always
reversible.

Not enough is known about other rare effects of danazol and
their reversibility. For example, one sufferer reported problems
with her contact lenses and then a drastic deterioration in her
eyesight, which her optican associated with fluid retention in her
eyeballs due to danazol. Fortunately, her sight returned to what
it was previously when she abandoned the tablets. This case was
dramatic enough to lead to use of the yellow card system,
whereby the doctor notifies the possible side effect (of any drug)
to the Committee on the Safety of Medicines. It may be more
difficult to convince your doctor to report a severe side effect if it
is chronic or a long-term aggravation of a previous complaint.

The Endometriosis Society followed up more than 300
women with persistent problems that might be related to
danazol treatment. The vast majority complained of joint
problems which developed while taking danazol, and in many
cases the joint pain did not improve when they stopped taking it.
It is not possible to conclude that danazol is responsible for this
effect on the basis of an informal study, but until further research
is done the findings do suggest it might be wise to choose another
drug treatment if you already suffer from joint pains, or change
to another drug if such problems develop.

Effectiveness

Whatever side effects you experience on danazol, you will want
to balance them against its benefits. So how effective is danazol?
It depends on how you judge success. For many sufferers it may
be having a much longed-for baby. Reports of pregnancy rates

after danazol treatment vary as the studies are not carried out in the same way; for example, different criteria are used for assessing how bad the endometriosis was, different treatment regimes are compared (e.g. sometimes surgery is performed as well) and different doses are given. To complicate findings, there may be additional reasons for a couple's infertility besides endometriosis (e.g. lack of ovulation, partner's low sperm count).

It is thus difficult to predict which women should have most hope of becoming pregnant. One summary of international studies reported that 31–53 per cent of those with mild endometriosis and 23–50 per cent of those with moderate endometriosis became pregnant after treatment with danazol. However, it is difficult to tell how many of these women would have become pregnant anyway without treatment (see Chapter 6). In general, women with mild endometriosis have a better chance of conceiving, but a few women with severe endometriosis have had some wonderful surprises.

I went for a laparoscopy and they told me I might not be able to have children. I was very upset. The endometriosis was extensive. I had to take danazol. After the treatment I was told I should try for a family. While on holiday in August realised I was pregnant! Our 10 lb son was born in April and I was over the moon. It was a difficult birth and they say the next one will be a caesarean, but I'm looking forward to it.

I was diagnosed as having widespread severe endometriosis after years of debilitating period pains. The endometriosis was found to be covering both ovaries, tubes, uterus, ligaments, bladder and in the pouch of Douglas. After the laparoscopy my gynaecologist told me it was the worst case of endometriosis he'd ever seen and that if my husband and I wanted children we should put our names down for adoption. He suggested I take 600 mg per day of danazol for six months. During these months my husband and I came to terms with the fact that we would probably never have children and rearranged our lives accordingly. To the delighted surprise of everyone concerned, I conceived just three weeks after ceasing the medication – a true miracle. [Doctors usually recommend waiting three months to give your body a chance to recover from the drug.] My daughter is now a typical four-year-old with a delightful little sister. I had a few side effects while taking danazol – about half-stone weight gain, stomach upsets and deepening of my voice which is the only effect that has remained. If I found the endometriosis had recurred I would have no hesitation in taking danazol again.

The next big question is does danazol help the pain? It is easier for researchers to find out how many women were able to get pregnant after taking danazol rather than recording subjective measures of pain. However, one American review says that danazol relieves pain in 90 per cent of patients. This finding has been echoed in other studies, although they have also shown it isn't a lasting relief for all women. But it may well do the trick for you.

Out of all the treatments I received, danazol was found to be the most effective. It was highly successful as far as I was concerned and for the first time in years I was totally without pain.

Recurrence

The pros and cons of danazol would be easier to weigh up if it worked once and for all. But this is where the term 'recurrence rate' enters the debate because, as one medical author put it, 'patients need to clearly understand that hormone therapy of endometriosis will not result in a "cure" of the disease'.

The chance of symptoms returning after danazol treatment varies from one woman to another. An often-quoted American study suggests that if symptoms do recur, this is more likely in the first year after treatment – 23 per cent recurrence, compared with 5 per cent and 9 per cent in the second and third years respectively. Another study indicates that recurrence may be higher amongst women who take a low dose (54 per cent recurrence in the first year after taking 100 mg/day).

A recurrence can be devastating, especially if pain was your main symptom.

Danazol for nine months. Pain completely gone. I could actually touch my toes for the first time in six years! Four months after stopping danazol, World War III broke out in my back! Returned to hospital for removal of left ovary. OK for another year. Gradually started feeling unwell – low backache, tiredness, heavy tender breasts, painful sex, trouble with bowels . . . danazol for eight months. Needed stronger dose (400 mg/day) to control and stop pain, which it did. Had problems with leg and muscle pains, so started taking water tablets [diuretics to reduce fluid retention] as well. Other side effects: weight gain, spotty, hair on head became very curly. Four months after stopping danazol, World War IV broke out in my back! Now control pain with alternative medicines.

Reading this story, one can understand how women end up taking danazol for far longer than initially planned. Little is known about the long-term effects of danazol, but even less is known about long-term use. Few cases are documented, yet some women contacting the Endometriosis Society have been on and off danazol for years in an effort to cope with their symptoms. No one should have to carry the burden of long-term hormones with unknown effects. If you are taking danazol long-term, recent recommendations are that your doctor should regularly take blood to test your liver function and blood fats (lipids). The first test is important because danazol causes the liver to produce extra proteins. The second test is thought necessary because danazol *may* increase the risk of coronary heart disease, especially in women who smoke, are overweight, get little exercise or have a family history of heart attacks. Some doctors feel that non-androgenic progestogens (the progestogens are the group of sex hormones that include progesterone, and non-androgenic means they do not have male effects), such as Duphaston or Provera (see page 45), are a better choice for long-term use because they affect blood fats less. However, it is doubtful whether long-term use of any of these dugs can be entirely justified. Often this situation arises because neither the doctor nor patient know what else to do.

Whether or not symptoms will recur after danazol is a hard question to face when you have spent months taking your tablets

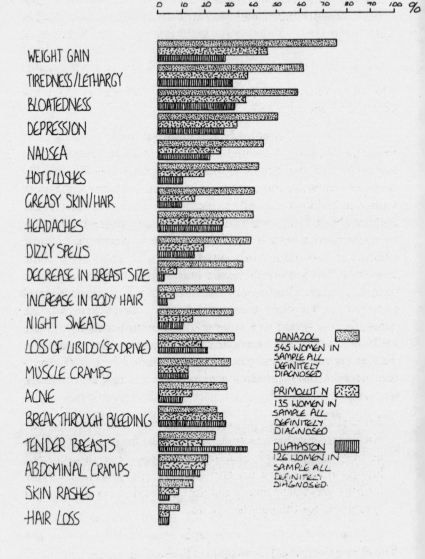

Side effects of drug treatment reported in the Endometriosis Society Survey.

in good faith. No wonder doctors (and authors) wish they had more answers. There is only one way to find out, and if you have problems, whether it be after a few months or ten years, you will have to reconsider your options. Facing this uncertainty and the knowledge that endometriosis is a chronic (long-term) disease arouses deep feelings which you may need to share (see Chapter 8).

PROGESTOGENS

The same precautions apply to this group of drugs as to the use of danazol (see page 38).

Primolut N and Duphaston

Primolut N (norethisterone) and Duphaston (dydrogesterone) are related to the female hormone progesterone. Technically they are known as progestogens, a general term for substances with effects like those of the natural hormone progesterone. Assuming you take a high enough dose, they stop your periods by tricking your body into a fake or 'pseudo-pregnancy'. These drugs are less commonly used (only 20 per cent in the Endometriosis Society survey had taken Primolut N and 20 per cent had taken Duphaston) but they may be a good second choice if you cannot get on with danazol. The side effects are generally less severe (see page 44), although progestogens are well-known for PMT-like side effects, e.g. bloating, irritability. Tender breasts are a particularly common problem on Duphaston. Breakthrough bleeding is also more of a problem than on danazol.

> After surgery I was put on danazol which had severe side effects, so my doctors suggested Duphaston instead. I kept getting breakthrough bleeding, even when I went up to the highest dose. I gave up and changed to Primolut N. Nine months' treatment finally did the trick and I have been free of symptoms for the past five years.

Provera

You may be surprised to be offered Provera (medroxyprogesterone acetate or MPA) if you have heard arguments surrounding the use of Depo-Provera as a long-term contraceptive in the

Third World or the debate about the risk of cancer. Provera is
the tablet form and does not have the same reputation for
leading to a delay in fertility after its use as the injectable Depo-
Provera. Some endometriosis sufferers have found Provera
helpful, where other drugs have failed. One study has shown
that a high dose of Provera (100 mg/day) is as effective in
reducing painful symptoms as 200 mg/day of danazol and that
both drugs were more effective than taking an inactive pill
(placebo, see page 73).

GnRH ANALOGUES

GnRH analogues (GnRHa) are a relatively new group of drugs
which get their name from **G**onadatrophin **R**eleasing **H**ormone
(GnRH). As its name suggests, GnRH causes the release of
gonadatrophins (e.g. FSH and LH) from the pituitary gland
which act on the gonads (ovaries in women). The drugs are
analogous (very similar) to GnRH so they can chemically key
into sites in the pituitary as if they were the GnRH. Molecules of
drug literally get in the way of real GnRH which would normally
tell the pituitary to release FSH and LH at the right time.
Without FSH and LH, the ovary won't have a message to release
oestrogen and the menstrual cycle will come to a halt (see
Chapter 1). This effect is known as 'medical oophorectomy'
because your body reacts as if the ovaries had been removed
(hence 'oophorectomy') but it can be reversed by stopping
treatment (hence 'medical' rather than 'surgical'). While you are
taking these drugs your body will have a reversible fake
menopause, with similar side effects to the real menopause.

Clinical trials on GnRH analogues have been going on in
several countries for some years and new members of this family
appear as drug companies develop their own versions. A lot of
work has been done on buserelin (marketed as Suprecur),
nafarelin (marketed as Synarel), goserelin (Zoladex) and leuprolide (Prostap SR) which are now licensed for endometriosis.
Other names you might come across, including histrelin and
tryptorelin, may only be available if you participate in clinical
trials.

GnRH analogues are often doctors' second choice of drug

treatment after danazol (and may remain so unless their relative costs improve). They tend to have far fewer side effects, although this will vary from woman to woman. Women usually experience hot flushes and more occasionally other menopausal symptoms, e.g. dry vagina with consequent pain during intercourse, loss of libido (interest in sex), headaches and depression. A small amount of bone loss can also occur (as it does after the menopause), but not enough to increase your chances of breaking a limb. All these symptoms disappear after treatment ends and most women replace the bone loss within six months. However, some doctors have doubts about using GnRH analogues for very lengthy or many repeated treatments of endometriosis because of this bone loss. Researchers are trying to prevent the problem by adding progestogen to the treatment. This certainly has the advantage of reducing hot flushes.

GnRH analogues cannot be taken in tablet form because they are broken down in your stomach, so you will be offered either a spray to sniff twice a day (e.g. leuprolide) or a small implant which slowly releases the drug placed under your abdominal skin (e.g. goserelin). There may be some irritation around the injection/implant site.

I'm 31 and have suffered abdominal pains and discomfort from a very early age. Other symptoms were nausea, tiredness, depression and a permanent feeling of lethargy – symptoms were so bad they were ruining my social and working life. I went to see a consultant who diagnosed endometriosis. I was offered a chance to participate in the buserelin trials. The drug is a nasal spray and very easy to use. I began to feel better almost immediately and my periods ceased after two months. Life became more meaningful and happy again. The only side effects were hot flushes and a few pains in my side. It is now four months since treatment finished and unfortunately a few symptoms have returned, although thankfully they are not nearly so severe.

I'd suffered from endometriosis, painful periods, ovulation pain and pain at other times for five years. After nine months on dydrogesterone (Duphaston), endometriosis was no better. I was put on goserelin (Zoladex), starting the third day of my period and given as a monthly injection of an implant just under the skin of the abdomen – a 'short sharp shock' which was soon over, sometimes leaving a small bruise. The first month I felt worse! Apparently the oestrogen level rises at first [Yes, this is, in fact, the case] so I had a painful cycle and a heavy period. Then the oestrogen level was suppressed and periods stopped completely – and hot flushes started. I had about 10–15 per day. I found it difficult to sleep at night. I had a slight weight gained of 4–5 lb but no other side effects. After six injections I was still having some pain. The hot flushes stopped six weeks after the last implant and periods returned two weeks after that. Six months later I am feeling much better but still have period and ovulation pain. I'd say it was worth having goserelin (Zoladex). Although I am a little disappointed with the result, it was better for me than surgery or danazol which were put to me as alternatives.

As these women's experiences suggest, some symptoms can return after treatment with GnRH analogues and in this respect they are no more effective than danazol, although in both cases the renewed symptoms may be easier to live with. For example, one study comparing danazol and leuprolide (Prostap SR) found that 57 per cent of women had painful periods again within a year, although 33 per cent found they weren't as bad as before the treatment. More encouragingly, 75 per cent found that pain during sex improved and stayed improved. Another study looking at danazol and nafarelin reported that approximately a fifth of women on either drug needed further treatment within a year. The recurrence rate for the other 80 per cent in the longer term remains to be seen but experience suggests it may be anything up to 15 years in women who continue to menstruate (usually older women who reach the menopause in this time will be relieved of their symptoms anyway).

As with most other drug treatment for endometriosis, you should not be pregnant or breastfeeding before using GnRH analogues. Barrier contraception should be used until after your first period (usually within four to 10 weeks depending on your treatment). If you are using a nasal spray and develop a cold, you can still use the drug effectively but avoid using a nasal decongestant for at least 30 minutes before (and after) and blow your nose well first.

GESTRINONE

Gestrinone (marketed as Dimetriose) is another new drug licensed for the treatment of endometriosis. It works in a similar way to danazol and has similar, although often less severe, side effects. Studies comparing the two drugs suggest that they both shrink patches of endometriosis and usually reduce painful symptoms. For example, painful periods were reduced from 75 per cent of cases to none; painful sex from 45 to 15 per cent and pelvic pain from 40 to 15 per cent on either drug. There was no significant difference in the rate at which painful symptoms returned on either drug: 57 per cent of the women who had taken gestrinone found their pain returned within the first year after treatment whereas 53 per cent of those on danazol had this experience.

As danazol was not suitable for me, my gynaecologist agreed to me taking gestrinone for six months with regular monthly check-ups. I found it much more bearable, although there were some side effects – a skin irritation which was worse at night, some weight gain on my arms and legs which seemed to become more muscular. My breasts became smaller and my legs and face became hairy. After treatment, I had a laparoscopy which showed no evidence of endometriosis, but now three years later I am once again seeing a gynaecologist with suspected endometriosis. Although I have suffered great pain, I am luckier than some women because I have two wonderful children, although at times they have been fed up with Mum not feeling well or being away in hospital.

Since gestrinone is more expensive than danazol and equally effective, you will probably be offered danazol in the first instance. However, if gestrinone is recommended you will only have to take it twice a week, usually in 2.5 or 5 mg doses, to prevent periods (although research suggests 1.25 mg may be just as effective). At first glance, this seems an improvement on taking tablets every day, but twice a week may be even more difficult to remember – even with a calendar pack! Like danazol, gestrinone can effect an unborn baby so doctors usually advise you start treatment after a period to ensure that you are not pregnant. It is not necessarily an effective contreceptive. Gestrinone should not be taken if you are breast-feeding and double check with your doctor if you are diabetic, are on anti-epileptic drugs or have heart, kidney or liver problems.

THE CONTRACEPTIVE PILL

It may be suggested that you try taking the pill continuously (rather than stopping for a few days between packets). Some gynaecologists regard this as rather dated or at least unsubstantiated advice. Studies that seemed to support this treatment have been criticised for not making appropriate comparisons with a control group. Women who have tried using the pill continuously for endometriosis often found that spotting was a problem and that severe symptoms remained.

There is some suggestion that using the contraceptive pill in the normal way (with breaks between packets) after other treatments may help prevent endometriosis returning in the longer term. This is based on evidence that endometriosis is less common amongst women who have used the pill for a long time. It is thought that lighter periods on the pill could mean less retrograde menstruation and therefore less endometriosis.

4

SURGICAL TREATMENTS

Endometriosis can cause problems which do not respond well to drug treatment, so your doctor may suggest major surgery of one sort or another, e.g. laparotomy, hysterectomy. In the near future lasers and other instruments adapted for use down a laparoscope could make major surgery less necessary.

This chapter looks at what operations you may be offered, although, as with drug treatments, the advice you receive will depend on your particular case of endometriosis and your gynaecologist, who will not necessarily be trained in the newer surgical techniques. This chapter also examines the issue of hormone replacement therapy after removal of the ovaries.

CONSERVATIVE SURGERY

In general, drug treatments have little effect on large patches of endometriosis or adhesions (scar tissue), so you will probably need surgery to remove them. If you still want to have children then conservative surgery will be recommended, which quite literally aims to 'conserve' your fertility. Conservative surgery is usually done during a laparotomy as discussed below, but other techniques such as laser surgery are available in some centres.

Laparotomy
A laparotomy is a major operation to open the abdomen compared to the quick look with a laparoscope. It involves about a week in hospital, followed by at least a six-week recovery period. The incision is usually below the bikini line and becomes more or less invisible once it has faded. Any ovarian

cysts (either blood-filled chocolate cysts or other fluid-filled cysts) and visible patches of endometriosis will be removed – unless, of course, this means removing an essential bit of you. Alternatively, the patches may be cauterised (heat-treated) in an effort to destroy them. The surgeon will usually try and separate adhesions holding one or both ovaries in the wrong place. This can bring dramatic relief from painful intercourse if the ovary has been stuck down and bumped at all the wrong moments.

> My doctor said I had a cyst the size of a hen's egg on my left ovary and recommended a laparotomy to remove it. They managed to free the ovary which was stuck down by adhesions between the uterus and bowel. I was amazed that my worst symptom, deep pain on intercourse, was gone! I was later put on danazol for remaining endometriosis.

You may have a ventro-suspension done at the same time, which involves tightening the round ligament although doctors disagree about whether this is worth doing since it is a feeble support at the best of times. Regular pelvic-floor exercises (see page 3) are probably far more effective.

There is no doubt that surgery is a good way to deal with large patches of endometriosis, remove cysts and separate adhesions in severe cases, but recurrences can still happen (28 per cent within 18 months and 40 per cent after nine years according to one review). There are several reasons why surgery will never be a complete answer to endometriosis. For a start, the surgeon will only be able to remove or cauterise what he or she can see. Endometriosis is often microscopic and the unusual forms or colours of the disease may not be recognised. Endometriosis may also be mistaken at times; for example, an ovary with a patch of endometriosis can look remarkably like an ovary bloodstained after a follicle has ruptured and released an egg.

Even if the surgeon is sure he or she can see endometriosis, it may be in a very delicate area such as near the bowel or ureters (tubes which carry urine from each kidney to your bladder), where the risks and consequences of accidental damage are too great. Equally, the chances are slim of separating a uterus stuck against the bowel by extensive adhesions without causing worse damage. Doctors often recommend a course of hormone treatment after a laparotomy to make sure that any endometriosis that is hidden or impossible to remove gets a dose of treatment. They may also suggest you take drugs before the operation to reduce the amount of endometriosis. This advice is more controversial with some gynaecologists questioning the value of suppressing patches of endometriosis and making then *more* difficult to see during surgery, only for them to return at a later date. Others argue drug treatment may shrink cysts making them easier to remove during laparoscopic surgery.

There is also a debate about the value of surgery to separate adhesions and 'tidy the pelvis up', as the operation itself could cause more adhesions. Obviously, incisions result in scar tissue as part of the body's normal healing process, and the peritoneum which lines most of the pelvic cavity (see page 3) is very sensitive to all kinds of disturbance; for example, there is considerable evidence that old-fashioned methods of operating, which involved handling the internal organs with gloves dusted inside with talcum powder, led to irritation of the peritoneum and build-up of adhesions. Newer surgical techniques aim to minimise damage to surrounding tissue and, hence, later adhesions.

Microsurgery

Microsurgical techniques are still rare amongst surgeons, so your gynaecologist may not have been introduced to them. Microsurgery requires special tools and meticulous procedures. For example, the organs are handled as gently as possible, using instruments rather than gloved hands. Metal instruments are Teflon-coated to give a non-stick surface to reduce abrasions, and smooth glass hooks are used instead of clamps and stay-sutures (stitches to keep things in place during the operation). Incisions are made using a microelectrical tool with a hot wire tip which seals as it cuts. Patches of endometriosis and small bleeding vessels are also sealed in this way. The area is constantly irrigated or washed with a special solution to rinse and cool treated tissues. Any debris is removed, along with the rinse, by suction. Care is taken to remove large pieces of tissue in one go rather than risk 'losing' bits which the body then has to clear up itself. Any stitching (e.g. to reshape the ovary after removing a cyst) is very precise and edges are folded in to make neat seams. Although these methods mean that the surgeon has to be very careful, methodical and even long-winded, they can have dramatic effects simply because the old adhesions have been separated and are not replaced with new ones.

If such care is not taken, the resulting problems with subsequent adhesions can be dramatic and debilitating. For example, Mary had a hysterectomy at 39, followed by removal of her ovaries a year later; though little endometriosis was evident at this time, extensive adhesions were noted by the surgeon. Endometriosis never bothered her again, but over the next few years problems with the accumulated adhesions really began.

The gastrointestinal pain gradually worsened. The diagnosis this time was duodenitis and hiatus hernia. Treatment did give a little relief but by January I was severely incapacitated and living on painkillers. At a laparoscopy no endometriosis was detected, but they found extensive adhesions on the bowel. My gynaecologist didn't want to operate as he felt major surgery would probably lead to even more adhesions within six months. He suggested that when I became bed-bound we would all have a rethink. I *was* virtually bedbound and unable to perform normal housework; walking upstairs was a nightmare. Persuaded by my friends in the self-help group, my husband and I sought an appointment with a microsurgeon through my GP. By now my GP was confused and baffled, but felt an appointment couldn't do any harm. The surgeon allowed us to explain the problem and then described his procedures. My impatience to get on with it were matched by his understandable desire to check for himself that the gastrointestinal problems were negative. After two months he was convinced, and I was admitted. When I surfaced from the anaesthetic all the pulling pain had gone and the surgeon left me with a lovely smile saying he was quietly confident. Ten weeks later I was doing things I had not done for years without pain – walking, gardening, making love and, best of all, picking up my grandchildren! A slow but sure invasion of my body by adhesions – all alleviated by a few hours of tedious surgery. Life at 51 is wonderful!

Laser laparoscopy

Imagine a high-energy beam of light that can be so accurately controlled it is possible to cut grooves in a human hair to a specified depth and you are imagining a laser. Lasers are an increasingly popular tool in gynaecology because of their ability to destroy tissue in a precise place with little damage to the surrounding area. Patches of endometriosis and adhesions can be 'zapped' and because treated tissue seals immediately with little bleeding, healing is faster with few adhesions. With experience, chocolate cysts can be drained and extracted and very delicate areas near the ureters or bowel can be treated. Furthermore, all this can be done down a laparascope (laser laparoscopy) avoiding the need for a major incision. Only two or three small incisions are made in the abdomen for the instruments, to aid visibility and to remove debris (and smoke!).

Laser laparoscopy has major advantages for the patient in terms of post-operative scarring, pain relief and length of time in hospital, but using this technique can pose problems for the gynaecologist and it is not yet widely available. Apart from the expensive equipment required, doctors must be well trained if it is to be used safely. According to one surgeon describing the technique, inexperienced doctors tend to find using a very powerful tool in a confined space where you can only see and feel indirectly is a bit like 'Star Wars in the pelvis'! Special operating procedures are required depending on the type of laser in use; one research paper describes almost mediaeval sounding measures to use a Nd-YAG laser safely: special goggles for all theatre staff, restricted entry and wooden shutters on the windows.

So is laser laparoscopy effective? If you have mild endometriosis, laser treatment is unlikely to improve your fertility any more than any other method or no treatment at all (see Chapter 6). Some doctors argue lasers can be very helpful in specific cases where the main problem is adhesions preventing the feathery end of the Fallopian tube capturing the egg released by the ovary. Laser treatment can also help restore the normal arrangement of your pelvic organs if your endometriosis is severe, but this doesn't guarantee your chances of pregnancy.

Initial research suggests that endometriosis doesn't come back at lasered sites, but in up to 50 per cent of cases it recurs at different sites – possibly ones that were not visible at the operation. This may account for the return of painful symptoms up to a year later in half the patients in one study. Comparative studies are being done to see whether laser treatment is more effective than no treatment at all; in other words, researchers are trying to assess how many women would get better *anyway* in order to see whether laser treatment increases this number (similar work is being done on drug treatment). So far it appears that after six months, 24 per cent of women improve after a 'sham' laser laparoscopy (where lasers weren't actually used) compared to 50 per cent who received treatment during the operation. If these results are repeated they might be explained by the fact that endometriosis is known to improve spontaneously (i.e. without treatment) in some women. It might also be true that having the 'attention' of a small operation improves some women's health some of the time (the placebo effect, see page 73)!

Some work has also been done to assess the use of lasers to block out various nerves to reduce pain – uterosacral-nerve ablation or presacral neurectomy. In general, this seems to be more effective for painful periods than other painful symptoms, but the results appear to wear off for some patients by a year later. Further work is being done.

Some members of the Endometriosis Society have seen laser treatment as a relatively quick and convenient way of 'buying time and relief' from painful symptoms even if, so far, it hasn't been shown to be more effective than many other treatments.

Angela was diagnosed when a chocolate cyst on her left ovary ruptured. She had a laparotomy and 'all the painful after-effects of such surgery'. Four months later, a scan revealed another cyst in the same place. She considered whether or not to have surgery again.

I decided to have the cyst removed whilst it was still fairly small as I could not bear the thought, or pain, of another rupture, and a bit of detective work led me to laser surgery. I was admitted as a day case and I was able to leave the hospital at 6 pm the same day. The whole experience was a lot less traumatic than previously. The laser was inserted through a half-inch cut in my abdomen, the adhesions burnt off, the cyst drained and burnt off as much as possible. Recuperation was a lot quicker than conventional surgery. I did suffer some pain for two weeks afterwards (where my cyst had been), but since then I have been pain free. The only reminder of the operation is a small scar.

Nicola also had severe endometriosis and problems with recurrent chocolate cysts.

My endometriosis was diagnosed and I had my left ovary and Fallopian tube removed. My main symptoms were severe pain, lethargy, heavy bleeding and severe PMT. Six years later (at 40) I was advised to have a total hysterectomy; my uterus was totally fixed and I had a large cyst in the pouch of Douglas. I was devastated. My GP was very supportive and tried to help me to come to terms with the situation psychologically. With my GP's and gynaecologist's approval, I went to see a consultant who agree to perform laser surgery. I had no discomfort immediately after surgery – not even from the three small incisions in my abdomen where the instruments went in. After a few days I did have severe pain before defaecation, which eventually settled down. I also had some side effects from the anaesthetic. I saw my usual gynaecologist six months later and he was very impressed with the improvement – my uterus is free again. As my endometriosis is still active I may have to have further laser surgery in the future. Meanwhile, my periods are far less severe and I have been able to avoid having a total hysterectomy and its complications at least for some time.

If you do opt for laser laparoscopy, you should be aware that a major incision may be required after all. This may be because your gynaecologist decides he or she cannot treat your endometriosis using this method once they have actually had a look inside or because very occasionally, accidental damage can occur which can only be repaired with open surgery. Further details on laser laparoscopy can be obtained from the Endometriosis Society (see useful addresses on page 163).

HYSTERECTOMY

If you do not wish to have children (or any more) and you are in your 30s or 40s, then your gynaecologist may recommend a hysterectomy, although women in their 20s with very severe cases of endometriosis have also been offered hysterectomies.

Hysterectomy means that your uterus and cervix will be removed (often referred to as Total Abdominal Hysterectomy and abbreviated to TAH). Your doctor may suggest your ovaries are removed (bilateral oophorectomy) at the same time, but this is a much bigger step than a hysterectomy. (See page 61). Do check with your doctor if you are not sure what is being recommended. Ask him or her to draw a diagram so that you know exactly what is planned.

The usual practice during a hysterectomy is to preserve the ovaries, but as one text puts it 'the question of whether to perform oophorectomy at the time of definitive surgery for endometriosis is difficult to answer'. If you are left with your ovaries (or one ovary, or even part of an ovary) after the operation, they will go on producing hormones, including oestrogen. If you have not reached the menopause, these hormones will ensure you continue with your menstrual cycles, so you may still feel PMT or familiar changes in breast tenderness, although obviously you won't have periods any more and you won't be able to get pregnant (even though you will be ovulating). The catch is that as long as you carry on producing oestrogen there is a chance that it will stimulate any remaining endometriosis. Patches may have been left behind, either because they weren't visible or they were on an important bit of you.

One review states that 'preservation of a normal ovary is associated with a 5–10 per cent chance of post-operative recurrence'. Another suggests this figure may be as high as 30–35 per cent in cases of severe endometriosis. You should be made aware of the risk before the operation to help you make your decision and avoid any nasty surprises.

Why was I left to work out the diagnosis for myself when symptoms returned almost two years later? I thought I'd gone mad as I'd had my hysterectomy and here I was with terrible 'period' pains.

It is even worse if you get a bad recurrence and your GP can't believe it either because he or she is not up to date.

One GP said my paralysing cyclical pain two years after hysterectomy (earlier appendectomy) was due to 'colic' and greeted it with heavy sarcasm: 'Well it's *not* your uterus, is it dear? And it's *not* your appendix, is it?'

In this case the woman had severe endometriosis and managed to get referred back to a gynaecologist who removed her ovaries (see below). If you are unlucky enough to get a recurrence, this may not be necessary; a six to nine month period of drug treatment may deal with the remaining endometriosis without the need for further surgery. Depending on your age, you may be able to keep your symptoms at bay until your natural menopause.

If you decide to have a hysterectomy, you will probably be in hospital for five to ten days. The operation can be done through an incision in your abdomen or, more rarely with endometriosis, through your vagina (check if you don't know which type is being suggested). An abdominal incision is usually horizontal, below the bikini line, but if you are overweight your gynaecologist may recommend a low vertical incision. If you have an existing abdominal scar, the operation will probably be done through the same place. A vaginal repair may be done during a vaginal hysterectomy to lift and strengthen support for the vaginal walls.

The usual advice on recovery from a hysterectomy is that you will need eight to 10 weeks. Guidelines on how long it will take to reach different stages of recovery abound in many of the books and leaflets on hysterectomy; they are useful for planning help with domestic work and/or sick leave, but such advice can also feel like a race which you are losing if your recovery doesn't go quite according to what is, after all, someone else's plan! Many women do recover in this time, but it can take much longer and a lot of women say that they weren't completely without aches and pains or extra tiredness for at least a year after the op.

Some controversy remains about whether or not hysterectomy leads to loss of libido (sex drive), changes in orgasm and depression. Research suggests that depression after hysterectomy may be linked to lack of discussion before the operation and lack of support by family and friends – which seems a natural reaction if you didn't get a proper chance to make your own decision and everyone expected you to get on with it and be right as rain in no time.

Whatever your feelings are, they are important – it is a big decision. You can't change your mind afterwards, in the way that you can if danazol doesn't suit you. The possible benefits of the operation need to be weighed against your endometriosis and your feelings. For some women the relief from pain where other treatments have failed or they did not get on with them has made it all worthwhile.

I took danazol for nine months, struggling with the side effets, but with little help for my symptoms. Things went from bad to worse and a hysterectomy was discussed. I had the operation, leaving my remaining tube and ovary. This all happened a year ago and I now feel the best I've felt for years and everyone tells me how well I look and I've loads of energy. I've gained a little weight, work part-time, garden and continue with my yoga. I've just finished painting the bungalow and am learning to swim! Hysterectomy (at 38) was the right decision *for me*.

Some women say freedom from contraception has done wonders for their sex life (although it should not be forgotten that barrier methods offer important protection against HIV). A few say their orgasms felt different but didn't disappear as they'd feared.

My orgasm definitely wasn't as intense, which upset me at first. A friend recommended pelvic floor exercises to strengthen the whole area and improve sensation, which I am trying.

Other women feel the loss of childbearing and an important part of their bodies, even if they were never desperate to have children.

For me the emotional shock was enormous. . . I did not really want children, but that did not make it easy for me. Not wanting and being unable are very different things.

I didn't want children, but neither did I want a hysterectomy.

If your endometriosis is mild and you are in your 40s, you may choose to wait until the menopause instead.

I didn't want to lose my uterus which had brought my four children into the world. I was also afraid a hysterectomy would affect my sex life. I asked for another opinion before making up my mind; the second gynaecologist didn't insist that hysterectomy was the only answer and agreed to give me annual check-ups. If I'd had cancer rather than endometriosis, I would have agreed to the op, but my endometriosis pain was manageable and I was willing to wait a year or two until the menopause. I have never regretted my decision.

Finding out more and talking to your doctor, partner and other women about the operation will help you make the decision. Ask for time if you need it. You can contact the Hysterectomy Support Network or the Endometriosis Society (see useful addresses on page 163).

REMOVING THE OVARIES

I know the medical profession have differing views on the subject of radical surgery. For instance, the consultant who performed the hysterectomy did not believe in removing the ovaries in someone of my age (I was 36 at the time) whereas Mr X believed that if a woman had severe endometriosis then the ovaries should be removed whatever her age.

Stopping the production of oestrogen by having your ovaries removed (bilateral oophorectomy) may seem the obvious way to deal with endometriosis once and for all, but there is a catch. If you do have your ovaries removed (either at hysterectomy or later), you will start to go through the menopause, whatever your age. This is because the menopause constitutes all the changes your body goes through when your ovaries stop working, either naturally or because they've been removed (surgical menopause). The main symptoms are hot flushes, night sweats and vaginal dryness, although you may experience a variety of other effects (see recommended reading on page 159 for books that give more detail). Long-term problems such as thinning of the vaginal walls (making sex uncomfortable) and osteoporosis (weak brittle bones) can also develop following the menopause and be serious. There is also an increased risk of heart disease. Doctors are able to prevent these changes by giving hormone replacement therapy (HRT).

My uterus, tubes and ovaries were removed. Symptoms remained but gradually became less and less severe. I consulted my doctor about vaginal dryness and was referred for possible HRT. I was given Premarin tablets for two and a half years. The symptoms did not return during treatment and I have not had them since.

The specialist recommended a hysterectomy which I decided to have. Unfortunately, I had to have both my ovaries out which was a terrifying thought at my age (36). He assured me that with a hormone implant I would feel like a new woman. He was right I must say that I feel wonderful. I have the implant twice a year. It sounds like a drastic solution, but it is a solution. I feel and think I look younger and it has improved my sex life.

Or you may prefer to investigate alternative approaches (see page 69). If you are deciding whether or not to have your ovaries removed and if you should have HRT or face a surgical menopause, you need to find out as much as possible. Reading around the subjects of the menopause, HRT and alternatives and talking to your doctor, partner and other women who have faced this problem can help you work out your options and what you feel about them (see useful addresses on page 163).

Hormone replacement therapy (HRT)

Hormone replacement therapy (HRT) is designed to replace enough of your natural hormones to prevent the symptoms of menopause. Most of the discussion you are likely to come across amongst other women or in magazines is about HRT for women who still have their uterus and therefore are given a combination of oestrogen and progesterone. Both hormones are given to prevent the slightly increased risk of endometrial cancer which occurs if oestrogen is given alone. Progesterone 'opposes' or balances the effects of oestrogen and so protects the endometrium. Of course, women who have had a hysterectomy (so no longer have an endometrium) can't develop endometrial cancer and can take oestrogen on its own. You will find women with endometriosis are usually on oestrogen-only HRT because they have had their uterus and ovaries removed (although see page 61). Their experience can be different to that of most women taking combined HRT as the commonly discussed side effects of combined HRT are often caused by progesterone.

HRT is available as tablets, an implant, patches or a gel for the skin. The treatment and advice you receive will depend on several things, apart from your gynaecologist's experience and preference. For example, HRT is not usually recommended for women with a history of cancer, but opinions vary about the risks associated with a history of blood clots or breast cysts. Your doctor may also think twice if you have problems such as epilepsy or liver, heart or kidney disease, or if you get migraines or are a heavy smoker. In some cases you may be told the benefits of taking HRT outweigh any risks. Do talk to your doctor about his or her reasoning if you are worried about being prescribed HRT, given your medical history.

The type and dose of HRT you are offered can also vary and

you and your doctor may have to experiment to find what suits you best. You may find that your gynaecologist intends to give you an implant immediately post-op to give you a chance to recover from the surgery before you explore different types of HRT; alternatively, you may prefer to start with tablets or a patch so that you can change easily if you have side effects such as nausea, bloatedness, tender breasts, headaches or skin irritation from the patches. In time, you will arrive at your personal preference depending on the side effects you experience (if any), practical problems and last but not least, how you *feel*:

I tried the patches but I do a lot of sport and felt self-conscious in the showers at the leisure centre. One day I had visions of my patch floating away in the jacuzzi! They also tend to fall off if you use a lot of body lotions after showering.

I didn't fancy taking tablets – it would be like facing the fact I'd lost my ovaries and was dependent on pills every day of my life. At least using the patch I only had to think about things twice a week.

I find the patches very easy to use but occasionally they are a real hassle – a bit of 'snapwrap' stuck on your backside doesn't do wonders in a passionate embrace and I suppose I'll have to give up fantasies about nude sun-bathing unless I want a teeny-weeny polka dot on my suntan! [the leaflets say you shouldn't expose that part to the sun anyway.] I might try the oestrogen gel which you rub in once a day, almost like a moisturiser. I hear it is very popular in France.

I started on Premarin 0.625 tablets but was constantly sick. Using tablets you need a higher dose of oestrogen because some gets lost [broken down by your stomach] before it reaches your blood. Using patches I didn't get nausea as the oestrogen went straight through my skin into my blood-stream.

I can get my implant put in at the GP surgery now which is much more convenient than the hospital. At least with an implant I don't have to think about my HRT much and having it replaced is no worse than going to the dentist.

The minimum recommended doses to prevent bone loss (and possible osteoporosis) are 0.625 mg of (conjugated) oestrogen or 2 mg oestradiol in tablet form of 50 mcg oestradiol in skin patches. However, younger women may find that a higher dose is needed to prevent hot flushes and other menopausal symptoms. Some preparations are easier to use if you and your doctor are trying to reduce the dose or use non-standard amounts. For example, Evorel patches are designed to be cut to size (hence dose) and tablets such as Harmogen are more easily broken in half.

Probably you will be advised to take the HRT continuously until you are of menopausal age, although increasingly doctors are recommending HRT for longer:

When my consultant discharged me from hospital he recommended that I stay on HRT until I'm 60. He commented that by then (in 24 years' time!), doctors may be recommending HRT until I'm 80!

The reason for this is doctors' concern about the increased risks of osteoporosis and heart disease in post-menopausal women generally and those who might have an early 'surgical' menopause in particular. This is a continuing area of research.

Another area of debate is whether or not oestrogen in HRT can reactivate endometriosis, so you may want to discuss with your doctor what can be done if this should occur. Many GPs will be surprised by such a question if they are not up to date on this possibility; some consultants would argue that it is unpublished, unproven or in any event unlikely. Research papers have been published reporting endometriosis returning in sufferers given HRT and medical advisors to the Endometriosis Society emphasise that the possibility should not be ruled out. There are no statistics to suggest how likely a such a recurrence is, but it is thought to be less likely than endometriosis being reactivated by leaving the ovaries in (see page 61). There is some suggestion that this may be because cyclical oestrogen from the ovaries is more likely to stimulate endometriosis than constant oestrogen levels produced by HRT. It is difficult to reach a conclusion on this when little long-term follow-up has been done. This lack of follow-up prompted one researcher at a recent symposium to comment he didn't dare try and answer the question 'is radical surgery and HRT the definitive answer to endometriosis?'.

The debate amongst gynaecologists about HRT reactivating endometriosis was reflected in the Endometriosis Society survey (although the advice women received was also influenced by their age). Sixty-one women (8 per cent of all replies) who had had their ovaries out were asked if HRT had been suggested. Just over half had been offered HRT, usually as tablets, whereas a quarter were told they couldn't have HRT because of the risk of reactivating endometriosis. HRT was not suggested to the remaining 25 per cent.

Some doctors suggest starting HRT several months after surgery in the hope that this will allow the endometriosis to 'dry up' first; others disagree:

> I asked my gynaecologist whether he thought a three-month gap after my complete hysterectomy would help avoid reactivating the endometriosis. He said in his experience young women losing their ovaries had such a miserable time with menopausal symptoms that it wasn't worth it compared to the very small risk of reactivating the disease.

> I had a complete hysterectomy. Two years after the operation I went on to HRT which I still take. I have had no recurrence of any previous trouble.

If your symptoms do return, you and your doctor can try experimenting with the type of HRT or the dose. By measuring your blood hormone levels, your GP will be able to assess how your body is responding to your HRT; this may help you both make a judgement about how much the dose can be reduced without endangering your health in other ways (e.g. osteoporosis).

Some gynaecologists recommend a preparation of oestrogen balanced either by progesterone or testosterone to reduce the chances of stimulating any remaining endometriosis, although again this is the subject of debate. (There is also some evidence that a testosterone implant can improve the loss of interest in sex, depression and lethargy which can be associated with the menopause.) Others argue that even if the endometriosis does come back, which is unlikely, at least you can stop the HRT for a while or adjust the dose. They may even advocate HRT on the grounds that it is easier to control than the oestrogen produced by the ovaries. This may be true in one sense, but the decision to remove two healthy ovaries and use HRT is not to be taken lightly while the long-term effects of this are not yet known:

If my consultant is right and I'm still on HRT when I'm 80 then I will be amongst the first generations of women to use HRT for 20, 30 perhaps even 40 plus years. Half my lifetime.

More research is required. Fortunately, this is an active area of interest amongst endometriosis researchers and those working on HRT in general.

SUFFERERS TALK ABOUT HRT

Age at op	Advantages	Disadvantages
38	HRT is very good for hot flushes and other problems if it can be taken.	My endometriosis returned and it took a long time to get back to feeling well again. I don't think I would take it again.
37	I started the HRT five days after my op and so in many ways continued feeling as before rather than menopausal, although I do get some vaginal dryness.	My skin patch irritates my skin unless I let the alcohol evaporate off before I put it on. I found the adhesive difficult to remove from my skin afterwards until someone recommended baby oil.

Age	Advantages	Disadvantages
36	General well-being, particularly my energy, skin and hair condition.	No one seems to know the long-term effects of HRT.
36	Protection against osteoporosis. No menopausal symptoms (i.e. flushing). Skin/hair not as oily. Even level of oestrogen with implant (no highs/lows) and can forget about it.	Slight risk of disease recurring. Slight worry about side effects (mild headaches). Not suited to everyone.
35	I persevere mainly because of an increased risk of osteoporosis. When I stopped for ten months I had bad sweats and faintness, which I am glad to be free of.	I hate taking tablets and I worry about recurrence. While off HRT I was free of arthritis in my fingers, but as soon as I restarted the pains and swellings came back.
31	In my case it is the only answer but I'm afraid it does not work for everyone.	The implants have to be inserted every six months in London. It's the loss of work for one day.
30	In many ways it keeps you feeling your age. After I had my ovaries removed I lost my sexual drive. At 30 this can affect your marriage drastically.	I have tried three types of HRT and at present use Estraderm 50 patches which seem to suit me.
27	As far as I am concerned HRT keeps me a balanced person. I have no side effects.	Although the implant is not a painful thing to have done, I resent the fact I am dependent on it. Even if I miss my implant by a couple of weeks I can tell the difference in myself.

27 I can't imagine why any-   The obvious one of bring-
    one would not want a   ing back the endometrio-
    controlled low dose of   sis. You must walk a
    oestrogen to stave off   tightrope all the time
    early menopause.   between too high and too
                                    low a dosage. Perhaps if
                                    you had your ovaries
                                    removed at near meno-
                                    pausal age, you would
                                    feel it more natural to go
                                    without HRT.

Alternative approached to HRT

If you agree to a bilateral oophorectomy but decide against
HRT, or are unlucky enough to get a recurrence of endometriosis when taking it, you may want to consider alternative ways of
alleviating the effects of a surgical menopause. There are many
books which describe what can help menopausal symptoms or
you may want to try suggestions from other sufferers.

I really did feel ill for ages after my ovaries were removed.
Then I embarked on the Ladycare range of vitamins for the
menopause. After two weeks the results were dramatic – no
flushes! I felt so much better, stronger and not so depressed.

I took HRT for six weeks and endometriosis returned. I heard
on a radio programme that royal jelly could be used for
problems of the menopause. I gave it a try and it works very
well. I take it with evening primrose oil. (See Chapter 5.)

I took *Agnus castus* (see Chapter 5) as a replacement for HRT
– burning feeling in body and headaches improved. I did not
expect it to clear symptoms, but it did!

I found that evening primrose oil relieves hot flushes and
makes me feel more comfortable. This took effect after two
months. Symptoms returned after I stopped taking it.

If your vagina gets dry, your doctor can prescribe vaginal oestrogen creams which can help enormously. Do not be tempted to use them as a lubricant during sex as they can be absorbed through your partner's skin too! A little vitamin E oil carefully rubbed into the vagina is an alternative to oestrogen cream.

Osteoporosis

Osteoporosis is a very common problem in women after the menopause because lack of oestrogen in some way seems to allow the calcium content of bone to be reduced, with the result that your skeleton becomes brittle and more likely to break. Many older women develop bent backs (and may actually shrink in height) because weak vertebrae in their spines become compressed and crumble. The Osteoporosis Society (see Useful Addresses on page 163) recommends ways of preventing this, including increasing calcium in your diet and regular exercise, although recent studies suggest that extra calcium may not be as protective as originally hoped. HRT is still the best way to prevent osteoporosis, but treatments based on other hormones such as calcitonin (which 'pushes' calcium from the blood into the bones) are being developed which may help if you can't take HRT.

I was 28 when I was told I had endometriosis. Eleven years later and some six laparoscopies, three laparotomies, one bout of laser treatment, a year of danazol, two lots of Zoladex, to say nothing of the pill, Primolut N or Duphaston – enough was enough. I had a complete hysterectomy. During all this time I built up my career and supported myself determined to prove I had this endometriosis thing under control. And for much of the time I did. Horrendous though this list sounds, each one bought me time – time from pain, time from interrupted nights, time to enjoy life.

As I got older the choices became fewer: repeated GnRH analogue treatment wasn't advisable, surgery was becoming more difficult with the build-up of adhesions. Hysterectomy was first mentioned, very gently, about three years before I finally went through with it. Despite the pain, it seemed too radical and final an option at first, and the various consultants I saw over this period, to their credit, never forced the issue. It was to be my choice, at my own time.

What changed my mind? One particularly nasty bout of pain which I couldn't fight any longer. I was unable to work and it almost ruined a holiday. In front stretched years of uncertain health and I didn't want any more of it. I deserved the best chance of health and freedom from pain and with that, I knew the time was right for the hysterectomy.

The post-op period has not been straightforward, even though two days after surgery I realised the constant grinding ovarian pain had gone. It has been difficult to balance the HRT; my memory was appalling for a time (but is now improving) and I certainly wasn't prepared for months of vaginal discharge. Regrets? No! Despite the setbacks, it was the right decision for me and at the right time. I daren't say it was the end of the road, because I get to the end and realise it's only a bend and the road still stretches ahead. That's endometriosis for you. But there's only one lifetime and I intend to give it my best shot.

I'd always had very painful periods as a teenager which my GP said were because I had 'a complex about being a woman'! If I met him now I'd say that having endometriosis is enough to give anyone a complex about being a woman! After all, it affects every aspect of your life as a woman – certainly how you feel and see yourself as a lover and possible mother or even as an everyday person who is or isn't able to work and play!

I was eventually diagnosed at 22 after sex had become painful as well. I had surgery and then drug treatment. Although I only had one ovary, after that I was fine and got on with life. By my early 30s I was beginning to think about having children, but my partner of 10 years 'met someone else' which was a terrible shock.

It was five years before I met David and we were in the midst of selling houses and planning to get married when I started spotting mid-cycle and having odd pains on my right side. These symptoms were so different from 14 years earlier it didn't really occur to me that it could be endometriosis again – although looking back I think I didn't really want to face the possibility. I delayed going to a GP until things were clearly getting worse. I had an ultrasound scan just before Easter – I remember all the Easter eggs in the shop windows as I tried to take in the fact they'd found two large cysts on my ovary. I saw a gynaecologist very quickly after that as the cysts were 12 cm across and I was bleeding almost continuously now. I couldn't believe my remaining ovary had probably been destroyed by the cysts and he was recommending a hysterectomy. I asked for a fortnight to make up my mind even though I was getting rapidly worse and in that time I realised that given my age and the mess I was in I had to go ahead.

Everyone – my family and my doctors – were superb but it has taken me a year to adjust. My endometriosis had come back with a vengeance and when they operated there was no chance of saving anything. However, I'm OK on HRT and life is looking good again. David and I have learnt a lot going through all this together and are still getting married – although a year later than planned thanks to my op!

I realise we were spared the repeated grief of trying for a child and as my doctor said we probably never stood a chance anyway. My sister had her second baby six weeks after my hysterectomy which was hard for both of us but I adore my two nieces and feel able to share in their lives, even if I've also shed many tears. Endometriosis eventually forced me into a very hard painful decision but I have also had 14 years without pain. Perhaps if I'd met the 'right' person in my 20s life would have been different, but I'm sure I'm not the only person in the world who has thought that!

5

ALTERNATIVE AND COMPLEMENTARY APPROACHES

This chapter is based on the experiences of endometriosis sufferers who have found help using different approaches to the orthodox treatments described in Chapters 3 and 4. Many have been able to relieve their symptoms; others feel they have found a complete cure. Sufferers often try alternative medicine when they feel drugs and surgery have not helped, but some have found therapies complementary to the treatment they are receiving.

A wide range of supplements, remedies and alternative approaches are briefly described. Do turn to the recommended reading and useful addresses lists if you want to investigate anything in more detail or contact a practitioner. Do not expect immediate results; many comments show that you need to allow at least a month or two before you give up. In some cases, you may find symptoms get worse initially. Alternative practitioners – like doctors – do not necessarily agree on the best approach to endometriosis, but this chapter will give you a starting point.

DO THEY WORK?

Many people report benefits from alternative approaches but there have been very few studies of their effectiveness (partly because of lack of research monies). A good test would be to compare the medicine with an inactive product (placebo) in a double-blind placebo-controlled trial. Unmarked pills are given, so neither researchers nor volunteers (double-blind) know who received what until afterwards. These sort of trials are important because they allow for the 'placebo effect'; research shows one would expect up to 30 per cent of patients taking the inactive pill to report improvements, so anything that is active should have even better results. No one knows why the placebo effect occurs but it may be to do with people's expectations that any treatment will help – an example of mind over matter.

Of course, few treatments, even those described in Chapters 3 and 4, have been tested in this way. Clinical trials for drugs tend to compare drugs with each other rather than with a placebo, simply because of the ethical problems of giving a patient inactive pills when this may not be in her best interests. Alternative practitioners will feel a similar obligation to treat someone with something they believe will help rather than do research on her. And there are ethical and practical problems in testing surgery in this way – surgeons cannot be blind to what they are doing, and cannot justify opening one patient up and treating her and opening another up and and not treating her for the sake of comparison. All this means the debate about what has been proven to be effective – whether orthodox or alternative – is complicated and that you will need to judge studies and individual experiences in this light. On the other hand, if you find something that works, you might not be too worried about whether or not it is the placebo effect as long as it lasts.

VITAMINS, MINERALS, OILS AND EXTRACTS

Sufferers have found various supplements relieve complaints such as premenstrual syndrome (PMS) and pain (also see Chapter 9). Supplements are expensive so you may prefer to use natural food sources wherever possible.

Vitamin B6 and vitamin B complex

In the early 1970s researchers reported the successful use of vitamin B6 to combat depression in women on the pill. More recent studies have demonstrated significant improvements in premenstrual symptoms in 50–60 per cent of patients on 80–100 mg per day. Vitamin B6 is now a popular home remedy for PMS and many GPs prescribe it.

The reasons why vitamin B6 should help PMS are still poorly

understood, but it appears to be important in the production of certain substances influencing the pituitary gland (and hence the menstrual cycle) and the production of other chemicals thought to regulate mood. Many endometriosis sufferers have found vitamin B6 helps PMS symptoms such as irritability and bloatedness which they report throughout the month, while others have found that it reduces side effects of hormone treatment, especially tiredness and depression.

The starting dose recommended for PMS is 50 mg of vitamin B6 twice a day with meals, increasing the dose if necessary. Megadosing (500 mg/day or more) in the USA highlighted the danger of nervous disorders which develop when you take too much vitamin B6. Up to 200 mg/day is said to be safe, although the maximum dose can cause stomach upsets. In addition to vitamin B6, 25–50 mg of vitamin B complex is often recommended, particularly if you are under a lot of stress, have problems eating a balanced diet or suffer from poor absorption, but you must note the dose of vitamin B6 in the complex tablet so you do not take too much altogether.

Brewer's yeast, wheatgerm, cabbage and eggs are amongst good sources of vitamin B6.

Evening primrose oil (EPO)

The American Indians used evening primrose oil (EPO) for asthma and skin disorders, but it has recently become popular for premenstrual symptoms. An open study (i.e. not blind) showed that 62 per cent of women with PMS, who had not responded to other treatments, showed an improvement with EPO (i.e. better than would be expected, taking into account the placebo effect). Out of 36 women who suffered very tender breasts, 26 found this symptom improved dramatically, especially if they also stopped drinking tea and coffee.

Evening primrose oil is an important source of gammalinolenic acid (GLA) which probably accounts for its effectiveness. GLA is an essential fatty acid which helps the body produce a hormone-like chemical called prostaglandin E_1 (PGE_1 for short). PGE_1 regulates several body functions thought to be involved in the development of PMS. There is also evidence that zinc, magnesium, vitamin C, niacin and vitamin B6 are needed as part of this process – experience at a London hospital suggests that taking these as supplements, or making the appropriate dietary improvements, increases the effectiveness of evening primrose oil for PMS, although a proper trail has not been done yet. Evening primrose oil also blocks overproduction of leukotrines, substances thought to be involved in certain types of pain which are not amenable to painkillers such as aspirin (which block prostaglandins, see Chapter 9).

More importantly in this context, endometriosis sufferers have also found evening primrose oil helpful.

Mood swings – improved within a month; adhesion pain – improved within two months; period cramps – slightly better.

Severe abdominal pain, difficulty in walking, dryness in vagina, all relieved within ten days of starting EPO.

I have been taking EPO for 18 months. I start on the 10th day of my cycle (3 or 4 x 500 mg daily). I no longer feel extreme tiredness and lethargy (some months I used to be too tired to go to work and had no energy for a social life). I used to have spots, cold sores and a very swollen stomach. My complexion is much healthier and friends keep remarking on how well I am looking. My periods used to be heavy, with painful bowel movements (endometriosis in bowel). I still have some pain, but nothing I cannot cope with, and only a faint show of bleeding from bowel. My GP was sceptical at first but he has since informed me that a local hospital had good results using EPO for breast cysts, and he now admits it could possibly have the same sort of effect with endometriosis. There have been months when I just haven't been able to afford EPO and all my past symptoms return within a few weeks. The only criticism I have is that my bust has grown from 34 to 36 inches, but that is a very small price to pay!

Sufferers have also found that evening primrose oil helps side effects of hormone treatments.

Side effects from danazol, e.g. muscle spasms and pains,

vanished completely with EPO but returned during the week's trial break I took. At present I take 800 mg/day of danazol and find EPO a great help in keeping the side effects at bay.

Look out for other preparations containing GLA, e.g. borage seed oil or glanolin from blackcurrent seeds. Cold-pressed safflower oil (10 ml twice daily) can be a cheaper way of taking GLA. Try a local healthfood shop.

Vitamin E

Vitamin E is recommended by some to help prevent thick scar formation and to maintain a healthy skin. Sufferers report that 600–1,000 international units (iu) per day helps pain which they associate with their adhesions. Vitamin E is also advised if you have fertility problems, on the basis that animals with vitamin E deficiency lose their fertility. However if you have high blood pressure and are on anticoagulent drugs, check with your doctor before taking vitamin E.

There is some debate about whether vitamin E affects oestrogen levels. Some argue that it regulates oestrogen and is beneficial; others warn that vitamin E may not be advisable if you have had your ovaries removed and do not want to run the risk of reactivating endometriosis. You will need to read round this subject before making up your mind.

Vitamin E is found in green vegetables, wholegrain cereals, soya beans and eggs.

Vitamin C

Vitamin C can help if you suffer from heavy bleeding; it strengthens blood-vessel walls and aids absorption of iron (a vital constituent of red blood cells), particularly if taken with bioflavonoids (for a time these were known as vitamin P). It can also promote healing after surgery. Some sufferers strongly recommend it for help with pain.

When I feel the inflammation from endometriosis increasing I step up my intake of vitamin C to 4–5 grams daily and within 24 hours there is a reduction in the inflammatory pain.

Selenium

Selenium is a trace element, i.e. it is essential for good health although only minute amounts are needed in the diet. Several animal studies have shown that selenium has useful anti-inflammatory effects and can improve the immune system, which could account for the benefits people report from taking it. For example, a Russian study on rabbits suggests that a combination of selenium and vitamin E leads to more antibody production in response to a vaccine than does selenium on its own, while open studies on patients indicate that selenium can help inflammation in rheumatic disease, and endometriosis sufferers report very positive results with symptoms of pain (although it may need time to act).

> There has been a steady improvement in pain over the past four months. I shall take selenium for the rest of my life quite happily and can hardly believe how much benefit I have had from it – in fact every bit as much improvement as when on danazol or Duphaston, which I was prescribed over the previous four years and which had such bad side effects.

> My symptoms diminished but danazol had a lot of side effects. As soon as I stopped taking it, the pain and diarrhoea started again. I was reluctant to have the remaining ovary removed and the consultant was reluctant to operate. However, after four months on selenium the pain is much relieved, the diarrhoea has stopped and I feel very much better in myself. The consultant is delighted. He is doing research into endometriosis and has asked me to send him any literature on selenium.

> Both the nagging pain on my right side and rundown feeling were much better after two to three weeks, and I feel much more able to cope with things.

Selenium is available commercially in several forms. Selenium ACE is based on yeast cultured with selenium, combined with vitamins A, C and E. Some authors suggest that a yeast (organic) base makes the selenium more effective (increases its bioavailability). If you are allergic to yeast or on an anti-candida diet (see page 92), selenium is available without yeast (check the label carefully). One or two side effects reported may be caused by a yeast base rather than the selenium itself.

I have had good results from selenium, but have had to give it up as it gives me fiendish indigestion.

The dose of a selenium ACE recommended by the makers is a capsule a day (i.e. 100 micrograms (µg) selenium), but endometriosis sufferers have used three times this dose without ill-effects. Onions and garlic, broccoli, tomatoes, wheatgerm and tuna are good sources of selenium.

Magnesium

Magnesium is important in the metabolism of linoleic acid (another of the essential fatty acids) and the prevention of PMS. Magnesium levels are much lower than normal in red blood cells of women with premenstrual syndrome, and were doubled after four weeks of 2 × 100 mg/day vitamin B6. Magnesium is also necessary for calcium and vitamin C metabolism.

Try a supplement of 300–400 mg/day (not to be taken after meals), or eating plenty of green leafy vegetables, grapefruit, figs, apples, almonds, nuts and seeds in your diet. You will be getting more magnesium if you live in a hard water area. Avoid diet drinks which contain phosphorus, which tends to block absorption of magnesium.

Taking magnesium with calcium in supplements such as dolomite, aids the absorption of both minerals (see below).

Calcium

Painful muscle spasms and period cramps have been attributed to low blood calcium levels occurring at the end of the menstrual cycle. Some sufferers have found a calcium preparation such as dolomite helps painful periods and joint pains associated with endometriosis.

I had joint pains in my knees for many years prior to dolomite and haven't had them since. I recommend six tablets daily.

Dairy products are well-known for their calcium content, but there are other ways of getting what you need without the fat in milk – dried beans, green vegetables, peanuts, walnuts, sunflower seeds and sardines are also good sources.

Zinc

Zinc is another mineral thought to be valuable in treatment of premenstrual syndrome, which is common amongst women with endometriosis. It also has other relevant benefits such as promoting healing and fertility. There are various zinc testers on the market which will help you find out if you are deficient. The recommended dose is 15–25 mg/day.

Good foods for zinc are eggs, herrings, oysters, wheatgerm, seeds and nuts. Avoid a lot of bran, which is said to prevent absorption.

Supplement 'cocktails'

Selecting what might help you from the above may be a bit daunting. The experiences of women writing in to the Endometriosis Society suggest that the following daily 'cocktail' of vitamins can be very helpful, either to help symptoms or to relieve the side effects of drug treatment.

- Up to 150 mg vitamin B6 with 50 mg vitamin B complex.
- 1–2 g vitamin C.
- 200–1,000 iu vitamin E.
- Up to 20,000 iu vitamin A.
- 6 tablets dolomite (calcium/magnesium).
- 10–30 mg zinc.
- 1 multivitamin/multimineral tablet.

Since last October I have been taking vitamin B6, 500 mg EPO and a good multivitamin daily. I feel a new woman and no longer have the feeling of complete exhaustion all the time.

Since beginning danazol in May I have been taking one multivitamin, 1 g vitamin C, 100 mg vitamin B6 with B complex, two selenium ACE daily. I believe that these helped to fight off the negative effects of danazol – I was out of vitamins for a number of weeks and there was a huge difference in my levels of energy.

Along with Primolut N (5 mg/daily) and selenium ACE (three tabs daily) I take many other vitamins which I believe all contribute to my much improved state of health.

I was 35 when I realised that conventional medicine alone was not going to be the answer to my future health. Armed with Mega B100, vitamin C, vitamin E, wild yam (a herbal anti-spasmodic) and the peppermint pill, plus a little fibregel, I was out of pain for the first time in years and able to eat almost anything painlessly.

You may prefer to try supplements one at a time instead, so you get an idea of what works for you – and avoid the expense of what does not. Or you can seek advice from an alternative practitioner who specialises in nutritional or vitamin therapies.

BIOCHEMIC TISSUE SALTS

I have suffered from insomnia and 'nervous tension' for many years. Kali Phos makes me sleep well, relax, feel calmer and more able to cope.

The Schussler system of biochemic medicine identifies 12 salts responsible for the way the body functions. Any problems are seen as an imbalance in one or more of these salts. Tissue salts are often prescribed by homoeopaths, but you can also try them yourself as they are available in health shops. You may find the following useful for certain problems:

- Kali Phos   for PMT and depression
- Calc Phos   for light periods
- Kali Phos, Silica   for heavy periods
- Nat Mur or Nat Sulph   for fluid retention
- Mag Phos   for painful periods
- Combination S salts   for menstrual nausea

The usual method of taking them is to dissolve them on your tongue with nothing to eat or drink and no teeth-cleaning in the next hour. Guidelines on dose are given on the container.

HERBAL MEDICINE

Herbs can be used in home remedies for various complaints as well as part of a regime prescribed by a herbalist. Some simple self-help methods are recommended for endometriosis sufferers by the Secretary of the National Institute of Medical Herbalists in the box below.

Treatment by a qualified herbalist can be very helpful for pain. The prescription recommended will depend on your case, but the tinctures (solutions of herbs) are bound to have lovely names, as well as offering help! A list of practitioners can be obtained from the National Institute of Medical Herbalists (see useful addresses).

SELF-HELP WITH HERBS

Pain	See page 146.
Tiredness, depression, irritability	Try herb teas to replace ordinary tea and coffe – peppermint or rosemary will invigorate, chamomile and limeflower will soothe and relax.
Tired headache	Try a mixture of essential oils of peppermint and lavender, one drop smeared on to the forehead (take care not to get it in the eyes).
Bladder pain, irritable bladder (where there is no infection)	Try meadowsweet tea, made like ordinary tea – one cupful (without milk) four times a day or as required. One batch can be prepared and kept in a flask or reheated, but a fresh batch should be made daily.

Digestive problems	Try ginger (see page 146). This can be used for flatulence or for colicky pains. Two slippery elm tablets chewed between meals can soothe – slippery elm has a healing action and is well tolerated. It can also counteract irritation of the stomach caused by some drugs.

I took tinctures of thyme, licorice black coloch, vitex, St Johnswort, motherwort and nettle – 15 drops on empty stomach three times a day. My healer also suggested hot and cold water treatments each day on my abdomen and a loose vegetarian diet involving raw veg and nuts. So far I have had two totally pain-free periods.

At present I am taking violet leaf tea three times a day. Ugh! After suffering black/brown periods for 16 months I have had the first (three day only – wow) red-blood period. Violet leaves are an exfoliant and wash out everything in the wrong place.

My menopause symptoms are controlled by herbal medicine. Unless something untoward is going on, I feel randy most of the time and I control my vaginal dryness with oestrogen creams. I have to have an extremely good diet otherwise things go haywire. Unless I look at the stress in my life and try and control it, symptoms return with a vengeance.

Vitex agnus castus

Agnus castus is a herb native to the Mediterranean, first recommended by the Egyptians for sexual disorders in women long before anyone knew about hormone imbalances. It is also known as chaste tree, reputedly because nuns used it to suppress sexual urges.

Research in Sweden suggests that *Agnus castus* affects hormones produced by the pituitary gland. Alternative practitioners recommend it for a variety of menstrual problems, including infertility. It is also said to be a mild antidepressant. Endometriosis sufferers have found it useful for various symptoms.

> Mood changes and cycle pain much improved.

> Greatly improved mood swings, depression and PMT.

Occasionally, though, people react badly to it.

> Did try taking *Agnus castus* but it gave me a headache, diarrhoea and made me feel dizzy, so I stopped taking them.

Agnus castus should NOT be used at the same time as hormone treatments.

Agnus castus is available commercially as an extract (it may be called agnolyt) or tablets. You may need to take it for several months until symptoms subside; then take it for a few further weeks. Some herbalists feel that you should only use *Agnus castus* under guidance.

HOMOEOPATHY

You might be forgiven for confusing herbal medicine and homoeopathy because the latter also uses remedies with exotic sounding names. However, homoeopathy is based on certain principles rather than certain medicines.

Homoeopathic principles were formulated 200 years ago by Samuel Hahnemann, a German physician who was disillusioned with 18th-century medicine which he saw as ineffective, with harmful, even lethal, side effects. He based his principles on years of methodical work testing his ideas.

One of the most important principles is the 'law of similars' – that the substance to cure symptoms is the one which causes temporary symptoms in healthy people. There are around 6,000 substances which qualify as homoeopathic remedies. Another principle dictates they should be prepared through a careful series of dilutions and shaking. Apart from making the solution harmless, this process is said to allow the substance to change from inert to dynamic; then it is seen more as an energy stimulating an organ's own self-healing powers. Many scientists argue that the solutions are so dilute that the original substance cannot still exist in it, but research published in the respected journal *Nature* (1988) suggests that dilution and shaking somehow 'imprints' the substance on water molecules long after the substance has been diluted out. So the debate is likely to continue.

Homoeopathic remedies can lead to symptoms worsening initially; indeed practitioners often expect to take a sufferer through past illness, and a resurgence is seen as bringing out deeper levels of complaint for treatment. This process is described by several endometriosis sufferers who found homoeopathy very helpful.

My very first remedy produced a terrible aggravation of symptoms, i.e. flooding and pain. However, my second remedy worked like a miracle and I had my first virtually painless and light period in years. From that point things began to improve. I suppose, honestly, I feel it has taken me four years of treatment before I was free of any endometriosis symptoms, and throughout those years homoeopathy has helped me to re-evaluate my life and ideals. It has also kindled a strong interest which I am pursuing on a full-time course in homoeopathy.

In desperation I went to a homoeopath. The treatment, sceptically begun, was dramatic. The remedy almost immediately made me iller than I had ever been, for about seven to ten days, but once through this phase I got better and better and was virtually symptom-free for three months. Then it began to get really interesting – my symptoms returned, but in a changed form. Apparently the remedy 'bumped into' glandular fever which I had when I was 16! My homoeopath treated the glandular fever and I have been getting steadily better. She is still working through the 'sludge' of past ailments, but I feel better than I have done for years. It has been difficult at times to stick with it, as 'reliving' symptoms is far from pleasant, but infinitely preferable to a bottle of tranquillisers!

Within six weeks a very depressed weepy, moody and very

unhappy person changed. I started to have energy, to live and enjoy life. The pain started to go and after a year I was feeling strong and very well. I still have little relapses when I am under a lot of stress and have allowed myself to become run down. I think the hardest part of alternative medicine was realising it works – its approach and theory is so different to mainstream medicine that I found it difficult to trust.

My first session was one hour devoted to me as a whole person, my history of health and illness, emotional behaviour and lifestyle. I came away with a changing perspective. I began to consider that it might be inevitable that I would develop a chronic illness because I had persistently failed to rest or ask for support during prolonged periods of stress, until I became ill. A month after this, all symptoms of endometriosis returned, almost as severely as ever. I continued with homoeopathy. My menstrual flow responded quickly to treatment (in my case pulsatilla). I am now five months pregnant and feel well and optimistic.

The third homoeopathic principle is to treat an individual's experience of symptoms rather than seeing them as part of an underlying disease.

For a reliable practitioner consult the Register of Homoeopaths available from the Society of Homoeopaths (see useful addresses).

AROMATHERAPY

Aromatherapy is based on the use of essential oils which typically have an 'aroma' or characteristic smell. They are known as essential oils because they are thought to contain, literally, the very essence of the plant from which they are extracted. Each oil is chosen for the specific effect it is thought to have on the body, but they may also be used in combination.

Essential oils have become popular home remedies, not least because they are relatively cheap and easy to use, readily available in health shops – and can smell divine! There are a variety of aromatherapy books available which suggest 'recipes' to help you devise your own aromatherapy treatment. Their general advice is to use four to seven drops of one or more essential oils, remembering that certain oils should *not* be used if you are pregnant and, with one or two exceptions, they should *not* be applied directly to the skin. The oil(s) can be added to a bath or made up with an appropriate massage oil using one drop of essential oil to every 3 ml of 'carrier' oil. They can also be inhaled from a tissue or used in a cold compress. Some books give advice on buying and caring for good quality oils. Alternatively, you can see an aromatherapist (see useful addresses) who will make a detailed assessment of your health and be able to give you specific guidance on the choice of oils and best way to apply them.

Aromatherapy can help women with endometriosis in a variety of ways. For example, one aromatherapy book (see recommended reading) suggests the following massage oil for your abdomen and hips as part of a treatment for endometriosis:

- Clary-sage   5 drops
- Rose Maroc*   5 drops   diluted in 30 ml vegetable oil
- Geranium   10 drops
- Nutmeg   10 drops

*Rose Maroc is unusually expensive for an essential oil.

Or you can use oils which encourage relaxation and pain relief, improve healing and scar formation or counteract infection after surgery.

> After my hysterectomy my aromatherapist gave me several massages to ease the aching in my lower back (I lay on my side!) and to generally help me recover. She used a made-up oil with lavender and juniper which relax and detoxify, and tea-tree to counteract the infection I'd developed. Sometimes she would use one or two other essential oils that were particularly useful for me; these might be different for other women. She also gave me an oil to take home and rub on my scar. It contained frankincense and lavender which are known for their rejuvenating qualities. I found rubbing the oil in a clockwise direction (the same direction as the bowel) was very soothing and eased some of the swelling. I still use five drops of lavender in my bath – it feels like a treat and helps me relax.

These suggestions are offered as guidance rather than for long-term use as many aromatherapists recommend varying the treatment oils after several weeks. Furthermore, do remember the skin is a surprisingly effective way of absorbing medication (see skin patches for hormone replacement therapy, page 63) and essential oils can have strong effects. They are definitely more than 'perfume'!

A MACROBIOTIC DIET

A macrobiotic diet is based on eating whole, unrefined foods – no meat, refined sugar or diary products. Cereal grains, beans, vegetables, fruits, seeds and seaweed, plus some fish and seafood are the staples. Those with a sweet tooth will be reassured by delicious desserts made with grain-based sweeteners (barley malt and rice syrup).

> I originally investigated the macrobiotic diet because from all reports it seemed to be the best way of improving the immune system and healing myself naturally without the use of drugs or surgery. My problems, apart from moderate endometriosis, included a small ovarian cyst, a fibroid and malfunctioning tube, so my chances of getting pregnant were pretty slim. In addition, I had low back pain, rectal cramp, pain during intercourse and a persistent leg pain, plus the unpleasant mental symptoms of depression and anxiety. After 20 months of adhering strictly to the diet, I brought my endometriosis under control and found myself pregnant (at 41!). The doctors, needless to say, were amazed!

> The dietary programme is restrictive but the cooking is straightforward and cookery classes are available at various macrobiotic centres throughout the country. Patience and determination are needed, but the results can be spectactular!

CANDIDA ALBICANS

American physicians interested in *Candida albicans* noticed that symptoms of endometriosis often improved with anti-candida treatment. *Candida albicans* is a microscopic organism related to the common yeasts used to make bread or alcohol. It takes up residence in the gut (from the mouth through to the anus), vagina and urethra soon after you are born. If you have had thrush, then you know it well – it's caused by the same organism.

A ROUGH GUIDE TO CANDIDIASIS

An alternative practitioner specialising in candida usually does an allergy test for yeast based on muscle function. Saying yes to many of these questions *may* indicate that you have a candida problem.

Drug usage

- Have you had lengthy, or repeated, courses of antibiotics (longer than eight weeks on end, or more than four short courses in one year)?
- Have you been treated for acne with antibiotics for more than one month continuously?
- Have you have steroid (hormonal) treatment?
- Have you had contraceptive medication for a year or more?
- Have you been pregnant more than once (this alters the hormonal balance in favour of candida)?
- Have you had a course of immunosuppressive drugs?

Symptoms

- Have you had persistent, or recurrent, cystitis, vaginitis, urethritis?
- Have you a history of pelvic inflammatory disease or endometriosis?
- Have you had recurrent thrush (oral or vaginal)?
- Have you had athlete's foot, or other fungal infections on the hands, nails, etc?
- Are you severely affected by exposure to fumes, pollutants, perfumes, etc?
- Do you have a variety of allergies?
- Do you suffer from abdominal bloating, distension and diarrhoea or constipation?
- Do you suffer from premenstrual syndrome?
- Are you lethargic, depressed, unnaturally fatigued?

- Do you suffer from poor memory or feelings of unreality?
- Do you crave sweet foods, bread or alcohol?
- Do you have unaccounted-for aches and pains?
- Do you have vaginal discharge and/or menstrual cramps?
- Do you suffer from lack of sexual desire?
- Do you frequently have spots before your eyes?

(Adapted from 'Your body's unwelcome guests' by Leon Chaitow, *Alternative Medicine Today*)

Normally, your body keeps colonies of candida under control but an upset in body chemistry or a weakened immune system can lead to growth getting out of hand, causing problems. For example, you may have noticed that you get thrush more frequently when you are on the pill or after taking antibiotics. Drugs which suppress the immune system can have a similar effect. Deficiencies in zinc, linoleic acid and vitamins B6 and C are also said to be associated with the proliferation of candida. People who are heavy smokers, drink a lot of tea and coffee and are under prolonged stress are likely to have a candida problem.

Thrush may be the most familiar sign of unchecked candida growth (candidiasis), but several authors have suggested that the yeast can also get into the bloodstream, causing a whole range of other symptoms. In this case they argue that candidiasis should be regarded as a systemic disease (i.e. affecting the body as a whole) and predict that problems will return if treatment is limited to localised measures such as use of vaginal creams/pessaries. No one knows whether systemic candida causes endometriosis or a weak immune system means you are likely to have both. Several sufferers have treated candidiasis themselves: others prefer to consult a alternative practitioner. This can be done while you are taking hormone treatments.

Treatment for candida

The treatment recommended by practitioners specialising in candidiasis has three stages: anti-fungal remedies which kill candida; supplements to restore 'friendly' bacteria in the bowel; and an anti-candida diet which discourages its regrowth, with vitamins and minerals to strengthen the immune system.

Medically qualified alternative practitioners can prescribe the fungicide Nystatin. The powder is preferable if you are on an anti-candida diet (see page 92) since the pills are sugar-coated. The powder can also be mixed with water and used as a mouthwash to treat or prevent oral thrush, before being swallowed. Other anti-fungal substances are available commercially.

- Caprylic acid –   very effective fungicide derived from coconut oil.
- Pau d'arco tea –   derived from the bark of an Argentinian tree and containing lapachol which acts as a fungicide. Other names include tahhebo, lapacho and ipe roxo. Pau d'arco teabags are available, or it can be taken in capsules or as a herbal extract.
- Organic garlic –   good anti-fungal agent. Take it as capsules if you prefer (e.g. kyolic).
- Chlorophyll –   toxic to candida. Available as a supplement.
- Homoeopathic remedy – your homoeopath may prescribe a dilution of candida or health shops may stock Nelson's candida dilution.

Many of the fungicides described above will destroy 'friendly' bowel bacteria as well, which you will need to replace. You may be surprised to learn you could have as much as 3–5 lb of bacteria to replace, but once colonies are re-started they should grow back again quite happily. Practitioners often recommend that you begin with *Lactobacillus bifido*, especially if you were not breastfed (a good source of this bacteria originally). Preparations include Vitaplex and Probion Bifidus. Then use Superdophilus, a very good source of *Lactobacillus acidophilus* (if you are allergic to milk use Primedophilus). Taking biotin (a B vitamin) is also said to be important because it stops candida converting into its more destructive form. Oleic acid (occurs in olive oil) also has this effect, so 300 micrograms of biotin are recommended three times a day with two tablespoons of olive oil. Restoring the balance can take one to six months depending on the severity of symptoms.

Anti-candida diet

The anti-candida diet is designed to starve existing candida and prevent its regrowth. It is seen as an essential step because you cannot expect to control candida while you continue to eat foods which contain sugar and yeast and so encourage its growth. Various books describe the diet in detail and cookery books will help you adjust your habits. There are still many things you can eat, such as fruit and vegetables, wholemeal cereals, certain grains, fish, eggs and organic meat.

Vitamins and mineral supplements are recommended to increase mucous linings (e.g. in the gut and vagina) to prevent candida passing into the bloodstream. They are also intended to strengthen the immune system so your body is better able to control candida colonies. Megadoses are recommended for therapy which are then reduced to maintenance doses, but you should consult a practitioner for advice, since people have different needs.

Drastic as treating candida sounds, some sufferers have had good results.

It is early days, but already the anti-candida regime has brought about great improvements. The first and most obvious change was loss of weight. Constant visits to the loo shed 17 lb of fluid in as many days! I found I had so much energy I drove my husband to distraction! I both looked and felt so much better. So far as the endometriosis is concerned, I am keeping my fingers crossed but my last two periods have been pain-free – altogether a miracle!

And several years later she writes:

I have now been pain-free for over three years. Periods are mostly clear and bright for approximately three days and often arrive without any prior warning whatsoever. I am on maintenance doses of vitamins which suit me, but no longer take beta carotene. I loosely observe the diet, although I still avoid bread and yeast foods generally. My main weakness is sugary foods and I do not always exert the self-discipline I should!

Dr X diagnosed candida and zinc deficiency by energy contact or muscle testing. She prescribed a yeast-and-sugar-free diet; apart from the obvious I had to cut out cheese, mushrooms, alcohol, chocolate, coffee and tea. I also had to take zinc orotate 100 mg three times a day. Miraculously, within five days my usual fuzzy head cleared and the pains in my stomach subsided. My energy level was about the same – tiring easily and needing a good eight hours at night and a cat nap during the day. After about 11 months on the diet, which after the initial shock I became quite used to (and with careful selection could manage to eat out on occasionally), Dr D said the candida was clear and I could introduce sugars again. I had lost 1½ stone, which was excess anyway. One tip worth mentioning about cooking is to introduce a variety of fresh or dried herbs to make the food more interesting.

6

ENDOMETRIOSIS AND INFERTILITY

by Caroline Hawkridge and Dr Stephen Kennedy

> For me the worst thing was not being able to have a baby. This has been the biggest disappointment in my life causing tremendous emotional distress. However, this is now behind me and I have learnt to come to terms with the situation, although there are times when I feel a bit down.

If you have just been diagnosed as having endometriosis and want to know if you will be able to have children, statistics and medical opinions are not easy to juggle. If you have a history of infertility you will want to know if treating your endometriosis will give you a better chance of conceiving.

This chapter will not provide all the answers, but it explains ways in which endometriosis could cause infertility and it discusses the merits of treatment options currently available. It also touches on sufferers' feelings about infertility and their experience of techniques such as in vitro fertilisation (IVF) and gamete intra-Fallopian transfer (GIFT). Several good books discuss being infertile in more detail (see recommended reading), or it may help you to get in touch with others through the Endometriosis Society or National Fertility Association (see useful addresses).

UNDERSTANDING THE POSSIBLE LINK

Endometriosis is associated with infertility – 30–70 per cent of women investigated for infertility are found to have endometriosis, and 30–40 per cent of sufferers cannot conceive. However, these figures do not necessarily mean that endometriosis *causes* infertility; particularly if the disease is mild. Mild endometriosis is quite common so some infertile women could have endometriosis by chance; likewise infertility is common, so some endometriosis sufferers may be infertile by chance. In the absence of evidence which explains how mild endometriosis causes infertility or how infertility causes endometriosis, the fact that they are both common in women may be coincidence. After all, blue eyes are common in women with endometriosis (and infertile women for that matter!) but this is assumed to be coincidental rather than related to the disease process.

Severe endometriosis destroys normal pelvic anatomy and so it is easy to see why it could cause infertility. A Fallopian tube stuck down by adhesions cannot pick up an egg and an egg cannot easily be released from an ovary containing large endometriotic (chocolate) cysts. This does not imply that you cannot become pregnant or there are no treatments which may help if you have severe endometriosis; pregnancy is possible, but it is best to be realistic about the problems that severe endometriosis causes and how they could prevent fertility. No one knows why endometriosis should become severe in some women and not others.

Mild endometriosis is defined as implants scattered on the peritoneum, without chocolate cysts or anatomical distortions caused by adhesions. Research into mild endometriosis as a possible cause of infertility has concentrated on three main areas – ovarian function, the peritoneal fluid and auto-immune response in endometriosis. These are complicated subjects in their own right; if you wish to pursue them, they are covered in more (rather technical) detail in medical texts on endometriosis (see recommended reading on page 159).

Ovarian function

A few women with mild endometriosis are anovulatory (they do not ovulate spontaneously), but so are many infertile women without endometriosis. However, treatment with drugs like Clomid, designed to make you ovulate, tend not to be successful in women with endometriosis until the disease itself is treated.

Luteinised unruptured follicle syndrome (LUFS) is said to be more common in women with endometriosis. This means that a follicle responds to the surge of lueinising hormone (LH) during the menstrual cycle (see Chapter 1) by preparing itself for ovulation, but fails to rupture; and of course, if the egg is not released conception cannot occur. Fertility measurements such as a mid-cycle body temperature rise and elevated progesterone levels in the second half of the cycle will suggest ovulation has occurred, but may be misleading because the egg is still trapped inside the follicle. Diagnosis can only be made by looking for the absence of a stigma (the hole made in the follicle by the release of the egg) during a laparoscopy or by repeated ultrasound measurements of follicle diameter – normally the follicle shrinks after ovulation, but this does not occur in women with LUFS. So many studies have reported a strong association between LUFS and endometriosis that some researchers have even suggested that LUFS is the cause of endometriosis, rather than the converse. However, more recently researchers have questioned whether LUFS is really demonstrated by signs such as the absense of stigma and suggested that further work needs to be done to assess how common it is in normal women.

Another reason why women with mild endometriosis may be infertile is that the corpus luteum (see Chapter 1) may not produce enough progesterone in the second half of the menstrual cycle, known as the luteal phase. This leads to short menstrual cycles and may mean that a fertilised egg cannot implant properly. Some research has reported luteal phase deficiency in endometriosis sufferers whereas other studies have found normal cycles.

Peritoneal fluid

The peritoneal fluid is the fluid bathing the pelvic organs. It normally contains a variety of different chemicals and roving cells such as the scavenger white blood cells known as macrophages. Researchers have been very interested in the unusually high levels of macrophages present in the peritoneal fluid of women with endometriosis and have suggested that this could reduce fertility in several ways.

Macrophages normally mop up foreign cells such as bacteria and sperm. Unusually high levels may result in sperm being gobbled up rather too enthusiastically, presenting a possible threat to fertility. Macrophages also produce several chemicals, including prostaglandins which help regulate muscle contractions in the Fallopian tubes. Some studies have found high levels of prostaglandins in women with endometriosis and argued that they could interfere with fertility by slowing down the Fallopian tube's contractions which normally help sperm to reach the egg. Alternatively, these levels could speed up movement of a fertilised egg so it arrives in the uterus before the best time to implant in the endometrium.

Other researchers disagree noting that there is no experimental evidence for these effects and that the stroking movements of cilia (hairs lining the Fallopian tube), which are not influenced by prostaglandins, are more important than tubal contractions. If prostaglandins do prevent conception then you might expect them to be effective contraceptives but studies have shown injections of prostaglandin-like chemicals don't prevent pregnancy. Yet another group of researchers has not found high levels of prostaglandins in women with endometriosis in the first place and so the debate continues!

Other chemicals in the peritoneal fluid of women with endometriosis are also being investigated and it is possible that drugs which counteract some of these chemicals may improve fertility for sufferers in the future. However, this research is still in its very early stages on animals and doesn't offer any immediate hope.

Auto-immune response

Chapter 2 described how endometriosis could be an auto-immune disease in which the body starts to attack itself for some unknown reason. To summarise briefly, current theory suggests that the body's immune (defence) system recognises endometriosis as 'foreign' endometrium because it is not in its normal place lining the womb. The body then responds by producing antibodies against its own endometrium (these are called auto-antibodies). These may be merely incidental to the disease, or they may contribute to the inflammation associated with endometriosis, as antibodies help in the destruction of cells (though usually the cells that are destroyed are invaders of the body, such as bacteria). Anti-endometrium antibodies are in the blood of many women with endometriosis and, interestingly, their numbers only fall in women who respond well to drug treatment. Some evidence suggests that the chances of pregnancy only improve in women whose auto-antibody levels fall after treatment, implying that auto-antibodies may interfere with conception and/or implantation.

So, does mild endometriosis cause infertility?

As you can see, there is no easy answer to the question of whether mild endometriosis causes infertility. The evidence is often unhelpful because it is difficult to distinguish between cause and effect; for example, all the disturbances outlined above can occur both in women with severe disease and in infertile women who do not have endometriosis. These disturbances could just as easily be major causes of infertility in their own right, rather than ways in which endometriosis adversely affects fertility.

If finding endometriosis during the investigation of many women with infertility is a coincidence, then this would help explain why endometriosis is also found in women who have never had any trouble conceiving. And it would also suggest that the results of endometriosis research which relies on volunteers with infertility (who attend hospitals more often and tend to be willing subjects) may not apply to other women with endometriosis who conceive easily.

Perhaps the strongest evidence against mild endometriosis as a cause of infertility comes from studies where women were randomly allocated either treatment or a placebo (an inactive pill, see page 73), without knowing which one they were taking. There was no difference in the number of women who got pregnant in either group. Therefore, 'expectant management' or merely waiting for conception to occur naturally, with the reassurance that it will with time, is being increasingly recommended to infertile couples where the only problem is mild endometriosis.

On balance, the evidence suggests that endometriosis is a cause of infertility, but it is difficult to judge individual cases. This is partly because present methods for assessing how severe endometriosis is are not sophisticated enough (see Chapter 2) and much more needs to be understood about what seem to be definite defects in the way the ovaries and the immune system work in women with endometriosis.

TREATMENTS

As suggested above, if you have mild endometriosis, you may not be given any treatment at all but rather advised to keep trying to get pregnant. In the past, many subfertile women with endometriosis were offered one of the drugs described in Chapter 3 on the grounds that this might prevent the disease getting worse. However several studies, including a big European project, have shown that women with mild endometriosis are just as likely to get pregnant with no treatment as with currently available drugs. Since you cannot try to get pregnant during drug treatment and it doesn't appear to improve your chances anyway, most researchers are arguing that there is nothing to be gained from taking tablets, when you could be trying for a baby instead. This advice makes even more sense when the drugs may have unpleasant side effects and probably only suppress the disease rather than halt it in many cases.

It has been estimated that approximately 20 per cent of women with mild endometriosis will conceive within a year without any treatment so this approach is increasingly recommended, especially for younger women. If you still haven't conceived after a year or are in your 30s when your fertility will be decreasing anyway then methods which actively assist fertility may be recommended to speed up the process (see page 100).

If, however, you have painful symptoms then you may be offered drug treatment to relieve the pain before you try to get pregnant. This could increase your chances of getting pregnant indirectly if pain was putting you off sex anyway. You may also be offered minor surgery, usually a laparoscopy during which patches of endometriosis will be cauterised (burnt away). Although this has been a common practice for many years, its value in improving fertility has never been established. Research studies have begun to address this problem but have been inconclusive so far. In some hospitals, cauterisation may be done at the first laparoscopy when endometriosis is diagnosed and be the only treatment offered.

The best hope of treating severe disease to improve fertility is to remove as much endometriosis and as many adhesions as possible and to restore the normal arrangement of your pelvic organs. As indicated in Chapter 4, surgery can be done during an open operation (laparotomy) or in some cases, down a laparoscope by a very skilled surgeon. Laparoscopic surgery appears more attractive if it is possible but its effects on recovery and length of stay in hospital are being debated. It may not reduce adhesions or treat the endometriosis any more effectively.

Summarising the success of the various treatments is an impossible task; claims for pregnancy rates following all these interventions range from 20–70 per cent, but studies are often not comparable because they are not done in the same way. Disease severity is often defined differently and the help of different sorts of patients is enlisted. Endometriosis may not be the only cause of the infertility being treated, and many studies only look at the problem with hindsight, which is a notoriously inaccurate way of conducting research.

FERTILITY DRUGS

Your doctor may suggest that you try fertility drugs, such as Clomid, to help you get pregnant. Clomid is best used to treat failure to ovulate; it makes the brain think oestrogen levels are low. The pituitary gland responds to these very low oestrogen levels by producing more FSH and LH, and sufferers often find their symptoms get worse temporarily as a result.

Several alternative medicines are said to improve fertility, including vitamin E, zinc and herbal extract vitex agnus castus (see Chapter 5). Women with endometriosis have also got pregnant after trying alternatives approaches such as homoeopathy.

IVF AND GIFT (ASSISTED CONCEPTION TECHNIQUES)

If treatment fails, or there is a coexisting problem such as your partner's poor sperm count, then you may be offered an assisted conception technique such as in vitro fertilisation (IVF) or gamete intra-Fallopian transfer (GIFT). In both cases, the idea is to stimulate the ovaries to produce a large number of eggs by giving daily injections of the gonadotrophins FSH and LH, contained in preparations such as Pergonal. Stimulation of the ovaries is monitored by measuring the diameters of the developing follicles with ultrasound, and when they have reached a certain maximum size an injection of human chorionic gonadotrophin (hCG) is given. This mimics the natural luteinising hormone (LH) surge in the menstrual cycle and helps the egg mature before ovulation. However, before ovulation can occur the eggs are gathered (harvested). At this stage the two techniques begin to differ.

With GIFT the eggs are collected during laparoscopy under general anaesthetic. A needle is inserted into each follicle and the fluid, containing the egg, is aspirated (sucked up). The three best eggs, with sperm, are transferred into the end of the Fallopian tube via a fine tube. The aim is for fertilisation to occur naturally in the Fallopian tube.

With IVF the eggs are either collected at laparoscopy, as described above, or using an ultrasound-directed technique that does not require a general anaesthetic. The easiest approach to the ovaries is via the vagina; an ultrasound probe placed there allows the ovaries to be 'seen' in great detail. A needle is then passed through the vaginal wall into the ovary to collect the eggs; most women are quite happy to undergo the procedure simply being sedated with Valium (to relax them) and pethidine (a painkiller). As many eggs as possible are then fertilised in the laboratory and, if embryos result, the best three are inserted into the uterus two days after being collected. Some clinics freeze any embryos remaining after IVF so they can be thawed out and inserted in later menstrual cycles. Equally, any extra eggs obtained with GIFT can be fertilised in the laboratory and the resultant embryos frozen for later use.

Many IVF units are now suppressing the hormonal activity of the pituitary gland with LHRH analogues (see page 46) before stimulating the ovaries with Pergonal. This yields more and better quality eggs, and also has the advantage of being a treatment for endometriosis at the same time.

Women with endometriosis tend to do well with IVF and

GIFT but if they have extensive ovarian disease there is a tendency for fewer follicles to grow. There is a debate, though, about whether IVF or GIFT is better for women with endometriosis. A review of data from American clinics suggested a success rate of 14 per cent per attempt for IVF and 25 per cent for GIFT amongst endometriosis sufferers. However, as GIFT is more appropriate for women with mild endometriosis this might account for the different results. The decision will partly depend on your partner's sperm, as there is a greater chance of fertilisation with IVF if the sperm are of poor quality. You must have at least one unblocked (patent) tube which is not stuck down with adhesions before you can have GIFT.

Success rates from the best clinics are very encouraging. However, the majority of couples entering treatment will not be successful. This uncertainty adds further stress to a very stressful form of treatment.

I have always had painful periods. However, three and a half years ago when we started trying for a baby, I found I had intermenstrual bleeding on and off during every cycle. My periods got heavier and heavier until that became more important to me than the gradual realisation that I might be infertile. One helpful doctor even suggested that it might be the excitement of a late marriage (age 27!) and the thought of a baby!!

To cut a very long story short, endometriosis was diagnosed by laparoscopy and I went into a nine-month-long nafarelin/danazol double blind trial (i.e. neither I nor my doctors knew what I was taking until after the research period). I was given Clomid almost as soon as I came off the trial. I had no side effects – only an almost overwhelming sense of hope at last. Indeed after four months on Clomid I did conceive, but sadly lost the 'pregnancy' two weeks later. We had been warned that the drug therapy would not cure the endometriosis and I might go back to square one and start intermenstrual bleeding again. I did not conceive again so we decided to try IVF.

The actual egg removal lasted an hour, there being 14 follicles. After four embryos were replaced, the waiting was rather stressful. We had been shown them on a video beforehand. I continually mentally monitored my body for any changes there might be. When the old familiar PMT symptoms came, it gradually dawned on me that it hadn't worked. It was worse for my husband. He thought of those embryos as 'babies' and he was sure it would work. I was not really optimistic but when you are desperate you are ready to try anything.

That was six months ago and we have recovered enough – financially and emotionally – to try again. We are going with less optimism this time, which I feel is the best way to approach IVF. It is easier to face the disappointment which, statistically, you are more likely to endure. If it doesn't work this time we will call it a day.

We are more at peace with ourselves now than we were after six months of 'trying'. It definitely starts to heal with time. Our friends have stopped trying to 'hide' new pregnancies which, in any case, never upset us. We have decided not to try and adopt – I think the process and the waiting would be much more traumatic than the IVF.

Endometriosis was diagnosed and danazol was prescribed for six months. After a second laparoscopy I was told I had three options: AID (artificial insemination with donor sperm), IVF and adoption. We decided to try IVF.

IVF is a very long process and tiring, but to reach fertilisation was good for us. But we were disappointed when a period started. Had we not applied to adopt I would most definitely have had a second attempt, despite the three week stay in London, and the Clomid and Pergonal injections, which were very painful.

As regards pregnancy, well I've almost accepted it may not happen – but we've been very lucky to adopt a little girl, Victoria, who was placed at seven weeks and is now two and a half. My infertility has been a great strain in my 14 years of marriage, but after being determined and trying every way to have a baby, adopting Victoria has brought us much happiness. One tends to put the eight years of tests and IVF down to experience – you were pleased to have attempted but only too glad to forget.

My endometriosis was discovered about three years ago but my consultant believes I've had it for about eight years, as I've had pain all that time and heavy periods. I took danazol for six months and suffered from terrible side effects and still had endometriosis afterwards. I wasn't prepared to take it for another six months and, as a last resort, tried IVF. The pregnancy was a difficult one. Things have not been trouble-free since but we are grateful for having such a lovely child. It does seem an absolute miracle that she is here at all. We would love another baby and plan another attempt at IVF, but fully appreciate how fortunate we are in having one baby. Life is so much brighter now that Miriam is here.

Of course, just planning to try IVF or GIFT can sometimes do the trick.

I came off danazol after 18 months and went on to Clomid to try for another pregnancy (lost first at 11 weeks). The heavy bleeding and severe pain came back almost immediately and it was not long before it was continuous. I went back to my gynaecologist and asked for a hysterectomy, as this seemed the only way out. He said I had one more chance which was a procedure called GIFT. After discussing this with my husband, we decided to give it a go. When the time came for our appointment, to our amazement I had gone over three weeks with no bleeding and was beginning to wonder if I was pregnant. I was pregnant – to the surprise and delight of everyone.

UNDERSTANDING YOUR FEELINGS

Both endometriosis and infertility are long-term problems and each woman has to find her own way of coping. Women often feel a sense of failure and that they have let their partners and families down.

Depression, frustration – I am a perfectionist. Guilt and sense of failure at inability to produce a baby.

I find it hardest to handle the infertility and depression and 'feeling less than useless' syndrome that are part and parcel of it.

They also describe grieving over the loss of a potential child. Other people's expectations or insensitivity, or a friend's pregnancy, can bring back powerful feelings of broodiness just when you are feeling more confident.

Feelings of grief, anxiety and depression (see Chapter 8) are a natural response to the problems endometriosis and infertility can bring, and many women feel in need of support when they are trying to deal with them. Turning to your partner can be problematic since he will be going through his own jumbled feelings. Apart from his own sense of loss, he may be finding it difficult to support you in your upset, anger or depression. He may resent pain affecting your sex life, the need to 'perform' according to your charts or the general change in your life together. He may feel you aren't recognising his need for support. It is well known that infertility can strain relationships, but the added problems of endometriosis can make it even more difficult to stay in touch with each other.

I had been hoping for another baby, but dreaded sex, which was often agonising, leaving me aching afterwards. This may have contributed to the breakdown of my marriage as my husband lost patience.

The main problem for me has been the effect it has had on my marriage. What other disease could be so socially unacceptable – or should I say sexually unacceptable? The symptoms are enormously stacked against a smooth-running happy relationship – long heavy painful periods, painful intercourse, permanent exhaustion, mood swings, constipation and, worst of all, infertility. The constant surgery, both minor and major, is extremely disruptive, and with the fear of total hysterectomy always just round the corner, it is very hard to relax and enjoy the everyday things in life which other women take for granted.

A husband writes a similar story.

My girlfriend became my wife in 1975 and about that time a
consultant diagnosed 'endo-something or other'. She looked
grotty for one week in every four, and often took to her bed
with a hot water bottle and the painkillers. In 1976 the
consultant said 'sorry, not much we can do, ever thought of a
hysterectomy?' Our world fell apart. Constant problems. One
week in four blacked out on the calendar – endless cancella-
tions, silly excuses. Love-making a disaster; painful for her,
and me full of fear of hurting her. In 1979 we knew we had a
fertility problem – tests, trials, drugs and charts. In 1984 we
couldn't take it any more – our marriage was almost on the
rocks, we stopped going to the NHS infertility clinic and gave
up hope of a family. However, we did go on a much-needed
holiday and then decided to have one more try. A new
approach, a new hope and as I write my wife is 12 weeks
pregnant. For the first time in 10 years we look forward to the
future together.

Turning to friends for support can also be difficult when most
people don't know what endometriosis is and find infertility
difficult to discuss. You may shy away from sharing your
feelings after a few embarrassed silences or too much 'advice'.
Attempts to protect you from their pregnancies can complicate
old friendships.

A very close friend had an abortion and didn't feel able to tell
me because of my endometriosis. I know she would have
before.

Many women (and their partners) have found that it helps to
share their feelings with others who have had similar experiences. This is possible through the Endometriosis Society or
National Fertility Association (ISSUE).

Since I had suffered from endometriosis for years before
deciding to have children, my infertility should have come as
no surprise: nevertheless, not becoming pregnant month after
month soon became the hardest thing of all to accept.

A sympathetic doctor told me about ISSUE, but at the time I threw his leaflet into a drawer. No organisation with such a depressing name could be for me, and anyway I wasn't childless; just not pregnant yet! Several operations later and still no baby and I hit rock-bottom. We decided to join ISSUE and it was the best thing we ever did. At last we had a group of friends – infertile men as well as women – who understood and shared our problems. If you're one of the one in seven couples who are childless (or just not pregnant yet!) please join us.

FOSTERING AND ADOPTION

Adoption can be a happy solution to infertility.

My new life free of pain made the knowledge of my almost certain infertility easier to accept. Never for one moment did I feel cheated, hurt or depressed. My only concern was that my husband would feel unable to adopt. My fears were groundless. His thoughts were for providing for a child already brought into the world who was in need of parents. We adopted twin girls at the age of eight days and they have enriched our lives greatly. There have been moments when we are reminded that they are adopted, e.g. mums talking about confinements and people commenting on how one looks like 'Dad', the other like 'Mum', but we have taken these things in our stride. Adoption can be easy to forget – our daughters are simply our daughters.

In some cases adoption may not be that simple. Rules govern who is allowed to adopt and nowadays not as many babies need adopting. The adoption procedure can be long and complicated and raise new doubts about your ability to be a parent – which no one will have questioned during infertility investigations. It will also require a lot of commitment from your partner. By contrast, it is relatively easy to become a foster parent. This can be a very worthwhile experience, but some people find it difficult to make a short-term commitment when they were prepared to make a lifelong one, and others feel concerned about the amount of involvement social services want with fostered children. For further details write to British Agencies for Fostering and Adopting (see useful addresses).

Becoming the parent of an adopted or fostered child can be an unexpected challenge when you don't have nine months' pregnancy to get used to the idea. You may also find it awkward being amongst other mothers (at last) and not being able to talk about pregnancy and childbirth. On the other hand, being able to share other pleasures and problems of having a young child will help you feel you belong. But be warned because adoption can have side effects!

I took Duphastion for 11 months, had another laparoscopy and was found to be clear. After that I took various fertility drugs which didn't work. However in June I found myself to be pregnant. I had a miscarriage and then a laparotomy which found a polycystic ovary and good old endometriosis. The endometriosis was removed and then I refused all other treatment for infertility. I just wanted to be left alone. In August we adopted seven-week-old Christopher. This was my best cure, I never felt better. However, in November we had a surprise – I found myself pregnant (no drugs or anything to help, only Christopher). Adopting Christopher was the best thing we ever did and because of him we are completing our family all in one year!

7

ENDOMETRIOSIS AND PREGNANCY

by Nicky Wesson

Once you are pregnant you are like other pregnant women, with all the same joys and sorrows. There are many books to help you, but if you have endometriosis you may have some additional questions and find it difficult to get answers. This chapter looks at whether pregnancy can help reduce the symptoms of endometriosis, and whether having endometriosis can affect your pregnancy or your baby.

THE DECISION TO BECOME PREGNANT

If you are young, do not have children and have severe endometriosis, you may be told of the risk of infertility (see Chapter 6) and advised to become pregnant earlier rather than later. Pregnancy may also be recommended to you as a 'hormone treatment' for endometriosis. While it is true that pregnancy can reduce symptoms of the disease for some women, the idea that it will cure every sufferer for good is an out-of-date medical myth. An Australian study showed that 40 per cent of those who became pregnant had no further problems, but symptoms returned in the remaining 60 per cent, usually within one to four years of pregnancy (just when you would be dealing with an active pre-school child). Other research work has been done since then which shows that pregnancy can affect actual endometriosis patches in several ways but in general, they appear to become less responsive to hormones during this time rather than withering away. This could explain why symptoms can return before long.

If you have a partner, want to have children together and are able to make the domestic and financial arrangements, you may be more than happy to have children sooner than you originally anticipated. On the other hand you may not be in this position, or you may feel that you do not want to be a mother and that changing your mind for the sake of 'treatment' is not good enough. Being confronted with the decision can be difficult.

I know they recommend pregnancy but it is just not possible at the moment. I do not feel ready to become a mother. But we are faced with a dilemma – do we wait until I am 30 and risk infertility or do we try soon when we do not really want to?

I was 22 and had just left university. It was hard to relate to what they said about the risk of infertility. I wasn't ready to settle down and my boyfriend didn't want kids. But when I saw a baby being born on TV, I burst into tears.

Although I want children, I feel to a certain extent I'm being pushed into it.

Even if your feelings about having children are fairly straightforward, they may be tinged with concern about your ability to conceive and carry the baby, and look after it if the endometriosis should return. If you do decide to get pregnant you can increase your chances of conceiving by making sure you (and your partner) are in good health. Good general advice is to stop smoking, gradually lose any extra weight, eat a healthy diet and reduce the amount of alcohol you drink. Various organisations provide further information about preconceptual care, e.g. Foresight (see useful addresses).

Some doctors suggest that you give your body a couple of months to get back to its normal menstrual cycle after drug treatment for endometriosis, before trying to conceive. This will not necessarily increase your chances of pregnancy, but at least your body will be back to normal before having to support a pregnancy. Sometimes ovulation can be delayed after hormone treatment, particularly with Primolut N and Provera, so you may want to take this into consideration when planning treatment in the hope of a subsequent pregnancy. Although endometriosis is associated with infertility in some women, many have got pregnant without any trouble, so do not be surprised if it works first time.

BEING PREGNANT

Little has been written about how endometriosis affects pregnancy, but some questions you may have might be answered by looking at two informal studies of sufferers who became pregnant. The first study, organised through the American Endometriosis Society, describes 187 out of 334 pregnances in 187 women. A smaller British study collected information about 100 pregnancies in fifty-five women (a few of these occurred before the endometriosis had been diagnosed).

At first you may be surprised by your feelings when you discover you are pregnant, and in this respect sufferers are no different from other women. Many in the two studies described feelings of delight, but others had mixed feelings; even women who have been trying for a long time can feel confused when they eventually conceive:

Tired, bloated and scared stiff at the thought of having a baby (11 years trying to conceive).

If you have been pinning everything on pregnancy, the reality may fall short of your ideal image; you may feel trapped, or worry about things going wrong. These feelings are common amongst women, with or without endometriosis, so it may help to talk to friends who have been pregnant.

Does endometriosis mean you are more likely to have complications during pregnancy? Early reports that endometriosis sufferers are more likely to have a miscarriage have proved unfounded. Several studies have been done on this and no significant difference in the miscarriage rate was recorded between women with endometriosis and other groups.

Bleeding during pregnancy can be a warning sign of a miscarriage, but 46 per cent of women in the British study had bleeding in the first four to five months which did not cause further problems. The bleeding ranged from spotting to heavy loss. This figure seems very high when compared to the 10 per cent for women in general in the first half of pregnancy. On the other hand, 16 reported bleeding without problems during the whole nine months in the American study. This suggests that bleeding during pregnancy may be more common amongst endometriosis sufferers, but need not be alarming. However, if you do suffer bleeding you should still check with your doctor at the time. Bed rest is often recommended, although there is no evidence that lack of rest is harmful.

You may experience unexpected pain during pregnancy – 54 per cent of the British women and 37 per cent of the American women complained of pelvic pain or cramping. Women in the British survey reported that pain often occurred in the early weeks, although some found it started later or lasted longer.

First three months very uncomfortable with lots of tummy pains due to adhesions being stretched.

Period-type aches in back and low abdomen and thigh aches for one to two months and at advanced pregnancy.

Considerable pain continues, sharp jagged pain all over.

All three pregnancies very uncomfortable and regularly quite painful. The first was the worst. I felt as though I was being stretched and torn inside my abdomen.

If stabbing pains are related to adhesions being stretched and separated by the changes in your uterus, they could even be beneficial! The surveys suggest that pain, often with bleeding, may be quite common without meaning anything is wrong – most women reporting these problems went on to have normal labours and healthy babies. However, to be sure you should contact your doctor. This is particularly important in the early months, as you may have an ectopic pregnancy (where the foetus starts to grow in the Fallopian tube, not the uterus) which is potentially very dangerous.

Of the British women, 33 per cent described the beneficial effects of pregnancy on their endometriosis pain.

Took several weeks for endometriosis pain to decrease, period pain – it was continuous but gone by eight to nine weeks.

Relief from endometriosis pain, PMT, mastitis [tender breasts], depression and irritability.

Total relief from endometriosis pain.

Wonderful relief, none of normal symptoms.

Of course, pregnancy also relieves premenstrual tension (PMT), which many sufferers report feeling during most of the month. This relief is probably temporary, as 59 per cent of those who suffered PMT before (67 per cent of British sample) found it was worse after the birth, 30 per cent felt there was no change and one or two felt it got better.

Far worse, two weeks before instead of a few days.

Yes, but much better, breasts not so painful, not so irritable, not so tearful.

Morning sickness is a less alarming problem which most women expect in the first three months of pregnancy, although studies estimate it only occurs in 30–50 per cent of pregnancies. However, 73 per cent of women in both the British and American studies reported nausea, which was often severe. In most cases, it had cleared by 14 weeks, although 12 British women suffered for most of the pregnancy. Nausea and vomiting were more common in first pregnancies. If this is a problem for you, alternative remedies can help and acupuncture before you conceive may prevent the problem. GPs do not usually recommend drug treatment; if your GP does, discuss any worries you may have about its effects on the baby and check whether the drugs you are given will make you drowsy.

Extreme tiredness was often reported in the studies, but this is very common in all pregnant women (especially in the first three months) so it is impossible to judge whether this is worse for endometriosis sufferers. Evening primrose oil can help relieve fatigue during pregnancy.

You may wonder about taking nutritional supplements during pregnancy. This is a controversial issue, so you may prefer merely to pay attention to getting vitamins and minerals in your diet. None of the vitamin and mineral supplements described in Chapter 5 are known to cause damage during pregnancy. However vitamin A should not be taken in doses above 7,500 iu daily as this can cause malformation. Sufferers have recommended zinc for severe headaches during pregnancy.

CHILDBIRTH

There is no particular reason to think that your labour will be any different because you have endometriosis. In the British study the length of labour varied from 31 hours to 25 minutes, with an average 11 hours, which is normal (taking into account that first labours are longer). Only three women had a caesarean section; two of these women felt the caesarean made their endometriosis symptoms worse, but a bigger study would be needed to find out if this was a common experience. A few cases of endometriosis in caesarean, amniocentesis or episiotomy scars have been documented in women who did not have a history of the disease previously.

Like women in general, women in the British survey often found labour very painful, but some felt it was easier to cope with than endometriosis pain.

Pain was bearable as, unlike endometriosis, you knew there was an end to it. I think that having endometriosis gives sufferers a much higher threshold of pain – I have found this in areas other than labour.

Women's experience of delivery varied, as one would expect, with 24 per cent having an induction, 18 per cent having forceps deliveries and 37 per cent having episiotomies. Some of these interventions were resented, particularly episiotomy. There are many books on childbirth to help you understand what you might be offered and decide what kind of birth you would prefer, given the opportunity. Talk to your doctors, your midwife, your partner and other women, and there are several organisations that can give you further information (see useful addresses). Antenatal classes teach breathing and pain-control techniques, which you may also find useful for endometriosis pain.

YOUR BABY

There is no reason to think that you will not have a healthy baby, but if you and your baby have problems you may worry that they are to do with your endometriosis or previous drug treatment.

Of the 60 babies recorded in the British survey, eight had some kind of abnormality. Most of these were minor and probably occurred at random. Fusion of the labia is the only condition that might be linked with drug treatment (see danazol in Chapter 3), although this has only been documented for women conceiving during treatment, not shortly afterwards. Surgical separation is possible.

Endometriosis does seem to run in some families (see Chapter 2), but long-term follow-up studies would be needed to find out how many daughters of endometriosis sufferers developed the disease. Current statistics suggest that your daughter probably will not get endometriosis, but if she does develop symptoms you can help her get prompt medical attention and make doctors aware of your history.

In the British study 55 per cent of the babies were described as having colic, where they cried painfully for long periods after feeding. This varied from a few days of mild colic to 'terrible' colic lasting for several months, well beyond the three months when colic is expected to end. There are no accepted guidelines about how common colic is, although one author comments that about 20 per cent of babies are generally expected to develop colic. The number of colicky babies in the British survey does seem comparatively high. Colic might be explained by a mother's *Candida albicans* infection (see Chapter 5) being passed on to the baby. If your baby is colicky or sleepless, there are organisations that give helpful advice (see useful addresses).

POSTNATAL DEPRESSION

It is normal to feel low a few days after having a baby, but 10–15 per cent of women also develop postnatal depression. This may develop gradually and can last months, even years. In the American study, 54 per cent felt depressed for eight weeks, on average. This high rate may be related to the number of problems experienced during pregnancy. Postnatal depression can be particularly hard if you have already struggled with infertility.

> I made such a fuss about wanting a baby, but now I feel depressed and exhausted all the time and I'm so irritable, even with the baby.

The unanticipated exhaustion and emotional upheaval of caring for a baby can be very difficult, even when a child is dearly wanted. If you feel depressed, talk to your GP or try out alternative remedies such as cranial osteopathy, homoeopathy and acupuncture which have helped some women. It can help a lot to talk to other women and get outside support (see useful addresses).

BREASTFEEDING

The majority of babies in both studies were breastfed – 83 per cent of American and 82 per cent of British babies. British babies were breastfed for an average of eight to nine months but most lactating mothers found that their periods returned before this at about four to five months (compared to mothers who bottlefed, whose periods usually returned within two months).

Breastfeeding is recommended generally for many reasons, but some sufferers have also wondered whether it could delay their periods and their endometriosis returning. An Australian study reported that 60 per cent of 84 sufferers had a recurrence within 1–12 years of childbirth, and concluded that lactation did not necessarily delay endometriosis. However, in the absence of further research, it is worth a try. Most women in the American and British studies who did get a recurrence did not get symptoms before their first period.

If you want to lower your oestrogen levels and delay your periods by breastfeeding, you do need to follow a few guidelines. These will help ensure that your prolactin (milk-producing hormone) levels do not drop too much, allowing a return to your normal menstrual cycle.

- Breastfeed frequently (intervals of less than seven hours overnight, and at every meal).
- Breastfeed on demand, including through the night (or wake the baby for a feed before you go to bed).
- Do not give supplementary bottles. Express milk for a feed if someone else gives the bottle.
- Introduce solids late (six months or more).
- Consider breastfeeding into the second year, i.e. after 12 months.
- Try not to be embarrassed about feeding your baby in front of other people. If they get embarrassed, that's their problem!

It is unlikely that you will need any of the drug treatments discussed in Chapter 3 while you are breastfeeding but neither should you be offered them as they can pass through breast milk.

CONCLUSIONS

The information about endometriosis and pregnancy is very limited and research with larger numbers of women would add to the informal American and British studies discussed in this chapter. There were wide variations in both studies, even within the experiences of pregnancy and babies in any one woman.

A few conclusions can be drawn through. If you have endometriosis, conceiving and carrying a pregnancy is not necessarily going to be difficult, although it may well be uncomfortable, with a risk of bleeding, nausea and vomiting. The labour is not necessarily going to be longer or more difficult than usual. The baby may well cry more or sleep less than others and you could experience postnatal depression. However, all these problems have medical treatments and alternative therapies. Vitamins and minerals may remedy some complaints. For those who get there, the outcome is felt to be well worthwhile – 'ecstatic', 'over the moon', 'worth it all'.

8
UNDERSTANDING
YOUR FEELINGS

by Lesley Misrahi

On days free from pain and discomfort I feel great and can cope with any situation. When I don't feel well, even answering the telephone is traumatic.

I found that as the endometriosis progressed I had mood swings, lots of tearfulness, feelings of insecurity, anger and depression which I attributed to hormone imbalance or disturbance which I saw as very much part of the illness.

The emotional aspects of a chronic disease such as endometriosis can outweigh your physical symptoms. Sufferers often feel heightened emotions in response to being unwell, undergoing treatment and the disruption of daily life. Many people would argue that this is a natural reaction to any illness, but many endometriosis sufferers believe that their feelings could be a direct physiological result of their illness. Premenstrual syndrome, postnatal and menopausal depression have been ascribed to hormone changes which affect emotional states. Since women with endometriosis may also have hormone imbalances, and the drug treatments for endometriosis alter the hormonal control of the menstrual cycle, it is not surprising that sufferers often report feelings such as irritability, tiredness and depression.

This chapter looks at the many feelings women with endometriosis can have and their need for emotional support as well as treatment of the disease. If you suffer from endometriosis, you will probably discover that you are not alone in some of your hopes and fears, and many women have found that sharing their feelings is a big step towards feeling better.

FEARS AND ANXIETIES

Fears and anxieties are probably the first feelings you can remember about your endometriosis. They naturally accompany the distressing symptoms and your not knowing what is wrong.

> I have always found not knowing the cause of the pain almost more difficult to bear than the pain itself.
> The worst thing about the whole time was the loneliness, the fear that I could actually cause such pains by neurosis and the final terror (subconscious at first) that I might have cancer.

Having a name for what you've got is often an enormous relief because it puts these fears to rest.

> I was so glad to realise I probably had a complaint with a name; it was something to go and investigate for myself.

Diagnosis is only the beginning, though. Endometriosis sufferers soon find there are other things to worry about.

> I am finding it all very frightening – the hormone treatment and its effects, the possibility of hysterectomy and, of course, the threat of infertility.

Fears and anxieties often arise from lack of information. Although information can give you more to worry about, in general people are more anxious about the unknown and what they don't understand. So finding out about endometriosis and its treatment may allay some of your concerns and help you assess your situation more realistically. Talking to people can help you to put things in perspective – realising that other sufferers share your anxieties may help you accept that these concerns are a natural part of coping with endometriosis. Some people are more prone to anxiety than others, and research in Belgium suggests that endometriosis sufferers may be amongst them. Talking to your doctor or gynaecologist (see Chapter 2) can help you take your anxieties into account when reaching decisions about treatment. For example, will you be better off having your ovaries removed if you are terrified of losing your femininity and sexual relationship, even if this does wonders for your endometriosis? Your fears need to be recognised and discussed before you reach a decision.

If anxiety starts taking over your life (e.g. with panic attacks), or crippling fear is preventing you from going for the surgery you need, your GP may be able to refer you to a clinical psychologist.

GRIEVING

When you learn you have endometriosis, you may grieve for lost hopes and expectations. It isn't easy to come to terms with the fact that endometriosis prevents you from doing some of the things that you want to do in life, or being the person that you want to be, such as becoming a mother or being someone who isn't ill, being a lover who isn't worried about pain on intercourse, or someone who has more energy for their job, family, friends and hobbies. Grieving is expressing your feelings about such lost opportunities.

Psychologists studying loss and ways of helping the bereaved have noticed that people often go through stages of grieving. Your feelings may not match these stages exactly, because endometriosis sufferers go through periods of hope and doubt (especially if they have to try a variety of treatments) rather than a single loss as in divorce or the death of a loved one.

Denial
I was unable to accept this had happened.

Imagine a situation in which you really feel like crying but are holding back the tears. All your attention is focused on not crying, so it is hard to concentrate on anything else. Are there any tears that you are holding back about endometriosis? What about your other feelings? You may have buried your feelings about the pain or infertility, to stop them overwhelming you and the other people that care about you.

Although this is a very common way of coping, it takes a huge amount of nervous energy to act as if 'everything's OK'. You may feel perpetually exhausted and unable to direct your energies to dealing with the disease.

> In some ways acting as if you haven't got a pain when you have is quite a lonely and estranging experience. My husband insists that I am honest with him about how I really am, and that helps a great deal.

You may be afraid that if you start to cry you won't be able to stop, but it can be very therapeutic.

> When I read the leaflet about endometriosis. I just sat and cried for ages. The grief was for all the years spent feeling that pain (particularly pain during and after sex, or being doubled up in agony on the bedroom floor during a period) was an inevitable part of being a woman and that to complain was wimpish, childish and probably a form of attention-seeking.

Denial of an illness can also take the form of unrealistic expectations. Often this is not helped by your doctor's reluctance to admit the limitations of current treatments (see Chapters 3 and 4) or the possibility of endometriosis returning before your menopause. Even if this has been explained, the natural tendency is to assume that your treatment will cure you and not to think until later about what you're going to do if it doesn't. Women have described how they felt unable to get on with their lives because they were waiting – to get better or to conceive, for example. Life improved when they reassessed their expectations and began to make decisions for the here and now, even if this meant accepting their limitations and finding new ways to manage.

> After several years of no social life, I hope to establish some nights out and see how I can cope with a normal life.

During these months my husband and I came to terms with the fact that we would probably never have children, and rearranged our lives accordingly.

Ironically, a perpetual search for the magic answer may get in the way of real healing. The classic example is when women find that accepting their infertility and making new plans suddenly does the trick.

My partner and I discussed yet another op, but decided against it – we started to plan our lives ahead without the patter of dainty feet. I decided that this 'thing' in my body, endometriosis, was going to stop ruling my life and I began to take control, relaxing more, learning to breathe and doing lots more exercise walking the dog than I'd ever done in my life. I began to feel alive again – and got pregnant! It was a shock to us both, and initially not really wanted. We'd mapped out a new life which didn't include a baby! But now our baby is wanted so much. I can't wait until July when it is due.

Withdrawal and isolation

Endometriosis often causes women problems which make them feel isolated or want to withdraw from people. Gynaecological complaints are not exactly an easy topic of conversation and most people have never heard of endometriosis. Your attempts to explain it may make you wish you hadn't bothered.

I thought that there was only me that suffered from this as no one had ever heard of it before. When they ask me what's wrong when I don't feel well and I try to explain, they look at me as though I'm silly. No one really knows what we go through.

People often react to someone who develops a chronic illness as they do when someone is bereaved. After initial sympathy and offers of help, they find it difficult to cope with their feelings and don't like to think of it going on and on. Lack of understanding gives them unrealistic expectations.

The trouble is, being treated in hospital, my boss and everyone else presumes I'm cured and so it is difficult explaining that it's always there.

Your response may be to withdraw from friendships and a social life. Endometriosis can also make you feel isolated in close relationships.

Endometriosis puts a severe strain on myself personally and my partner. This is due to changes of mood, lack of sex drive, tiredness and the constant threat of things being spoilt by pain. I feel that since the illness I have become much more withdrawn.

It is only natural to feel sorry for yourself at times, but if you find you are 'enjoying' sitting alone listening to sad music or dwelling on things that have happened to you (yes, other people have done it too!), then it's time to find support (see page 134 and the list of useful addresses).

Anger

Endometriosis can give you plenty to be angry about. You may feel it has ruined your sex life, made your job a struggle or impossible, prevented you from having children or made coping with relationships difficult. Your symptoms may have dragged on in spite of your remembering to take tablets for nine months or having major surgery. Anger about your life is a natural, positive reaction.

Even if it happens to other women, it still affects *my* life, creating tension and unhappiness in my marriage.

You have every reason to be angry about this suffering, yet many women find anger a particularly hard emotion to express. They go through cycles of feeling extremely irritable and then guilty because they have taken it out on other people.

My biggest regret as a result of this disease is the way I have treated my children. I shout very loudly when I should be calmly explaining what they are doing.

Family fed up with mother's moans, husband living like a
monk, tempers and tears, etc.

Paradoxically, it makes sense to take your feelings out on those
you love, because they are least likely to reject you for doing it,
but cracks may begin to show in relationships if this carries on
for too long.

The constant pain for months made me irritable. My
marriage was threatened for a while as my husband was
unable to understand why I was a permanent 'cross patch'.

Your partner may also feel frustrated by the disease continuing
and your perpetual need for support, which may not be
forthcoming after a while, unless you give yourselves a chance.

We both like walking, and this can be a very good way of
relaxing and leaving your troubles behind. It also gives you a
chance to talk.

If you seek outside help (see pages 132–6) invite your husband or
partner to get support for the difficulties he has living with the
disease too.

Unexpressed anger can turn into self-destructive feelings of
depression.

Felt diagnosis was very slow and spent a long time convincing
male doctors that I had a gynaecological problem (after first
laparoscopy showed nothing). Was given all kinds of irrelevant tests and felt very low about this.

No, it isn't easy to express your anger at doctors (see Chapter 2),
but if you are clear and assertive at least you know that you've
done what you can to improve communication. If you feel that a
doctor didn't diagnose endometriosis or warn you of side effects
during drug treatment, then try writing a letter. Perhaps you
won't send it, but writing it all down will help. And who knows,
if you do write and tell doctors the final diagnosis or the benefits
of knowing what side effects to expect, it could help the future
patients.

If you feel like shouting at God or fate for letting you get endometriosis, then let your feelings out – God is perhaps the only one big enough to take everything you can throw at Him without giving up on you. Or you can scrub the floor vigorously or knead bread instead. Or try this bioenergetics exercise, perhaps with someone safe around to support and encourage you: make a big pile of cushions and kneel in front of it. Take a deep breath in as you raise your fists over your head and then shout as you bring your fists down on the cushions. Repeat until you feel better.

Endometriosis can give you enough feelings of anger to deal with without taking in any more. So if bureaucrats, shop-workers or queue-jumpers annoy you, let them know as calmly as possible. Similarly, try to confront friends and colleagues as constructively as possible with grievances against them. Assertiveness techniques can help a great deal (see recommended reading).

Guilt and blaming

No one knows what causes endometriosis. If you have heard people use expressions like 'career woman's disease' (see page 31), you may blame yourself for not having had children earlier, without realising that there is no evidence that women who delay childbearing in favour of their jobs are more susceptible to endometriosis. Or you may feel it is your fault you did not get an earlier diagnosis.

I deeply regret not being more assertive when possibly an earlier diagnosis could have been made. I just accepted that I was over-sensitive to pain. I was my own worst enemy.

It is easy to get into a vicious circle, where you feel a victim and blame yourself for causing or contributing to the disease and then feel guilty about the feelings.

At the beginning of my illness I became very depressed, insular and moody. This generates a feeling of constant worry and guilt because it sorely affects what I, or my partner and I, can do.

'Don't blame yourself' is easier said than done, but it can help if you assume responsibility only for things you can actually change now. Perhaps you think you shouldn't have used the coil. Were you under too much stress, or eating the wrong foods? Until more is known about endometriosis, you won't know the answers, and perhaps not even then.

And say you found out using the coil was a cause. Blaming yourself after the event will not help. Being more assertive might have led to an earlier diagnosis (you don't know), but you did what you could at the time and it is difficult to judge how serious symptoms are and how much to push your doctor.

Depression
Everything is just too much trouble.

There have been times recently when I wished myself in heaven.

Depression seems to be very common amongst endometriosis sufferers. In the Endometriosis Society survey, 63 per cent said that depression was a symptom of their endometriosis (see page 13). Comments suggested that many respondents felt depressed because problems seemed out of their control.

I think I become depressed because I experience a lot of pain and see no hope of a cure. Also I am depressed by my inability to have a normal sex life.

Feeling very helpless because of lack of treatment and disinterest of doctors. Every day is the same, with no relief from pain and no pleasure because of pain and tiredness.

Equally, others have described how much regaining control helped their feelings and physical symptoms, through finding out more, meeting others, making decisions positively, trying alternative approaches, or adopting a new lifestyle (see Chapters 5 and 9). Remember you are just as likely as anyone else to suffer from premenstrual syndrome, postnatal depression, weepiness after surgery, menopausal depression (see recommended reading and useful addresses for help) and the commonplace ups and downs of everyday life.

Depression in fact can range from a relatively mild feeling of being 'down' to a condition which affects every aspect of life and becomes a threat to your well-being.

I am completely unable to enjoy life in any way. I neither laugh nor cry, I have no feelings at all – I feel like a robot. I am worried and forgetful and sometimes my mind literally goes blank.

If you have feelings like these and experienced a change of appetite and early waking or lethargy, you could well be suffering from clinical depression. You may also find that you start to use (or use more) alcohol, sleeping pills, tranquillisers or other drugs to help you cope.

If the depression gets to a point where it is having a damaging effect on your work, your family or your life in general, or if you are having suicidal thoughts, do go and see your GP before things get any worse. A short course of anti-depressant drugs may relieve the situation. It may also be possible to get counselling or psychotherapy on the NHS (see page 135).

Acceptance and resolution

Acceptance is the final stage of grieving. No one would suggest that acceptance after bereavement means that you forget the loved one or stop caring that he or she died. Similarly coming to terms with endometriosis is slowly accepting that you have the disease, that it may or may not get better or worse, that it limits you in several ways, but that it is not the whole of life and there are still many joys and achievements open to you, including some you have not yet considered (e.g. making new friends through a self-help group). When you come to terms with endometriosis you begin to feel better physically and emotionally.

For me the worst thing was not being able to have a baby. This has been the biggest disappointment of my life, causing tremendous distress throughout the years. However, this is now behind me and I have learnt to come to terms with this situation, although there are times when I feel a bit down.

I think we can only get better at the point where we stop asking 'them' to cure us and take responsibility for ourselves. That's quite a burden and in my case it was autogenic training (see page 154) that helped me take it on. I've still got endometriosis, but I'm not being destroyed by it.

If the idea of acceptance seems utterly impossible to you, you are probably still battling through other feelings. Coping with endometriosis is not an easy matter, nor is it a once-and-for-all thing. A recurrence of pain, or a sister or friend having a baby, can cause setbacks, upsetting the equilibrium you had reached.

CHICKEN OR EGG?

I sometimes feel I reacted emotionally to situations in my life because I felt so unwell. On the other hand it could be that emotional stress worsened, aggravated and possibly caused the endometriosis.

Researchers in Belgium, the United States and Britain are now becoming interested in the connection between endometriosis and emotional states and the possibility that stress contributes to its development. Sufferers often describe problems in childhood or traumatic life events before their endometriosis began.

My first husband left me in May 1975. Up to that time my periods were absolutely normal and like clockwork. From that date I went through a traumatic period. I met my second husband in August 1975, we married in 1977 and it was approximately six months later that the symptoms began.

Of course, everyone goes through a lot of problems so it may just be that there is always something you can pinpoint before your endometriosis started. However, research suggests that stress can upset the unconscious parts of the brain which control the hormone (endocrine) and defence (immune) systems. There is increasing evidence that disorder in the immune system allows endometriosis to develop and that imbalanced hormones assist its growth (see Chapter 2).

It is too early to conclude from research that emotional states contribute to or cause endometriosis, but the experience of sufferers does suggest that dealing with emotional problems and other stresses can reduce physical symptoms of the disease and encourage positive feelings.

HELPING YOURSELF

Find out as much as possible
I feel I could face up to the condition better if I had more information about the outcome of different options.

The relief at finding an explanation was enormous.

Most sufferers want to know more about endometriosis and its treatment. Reading this book is a good start! Plenty of information exists on related issues, such as infertility, having a hysterectomy, going through the menopause or alternative treatments (see recommended reading and useful addresses). The Endometriosis Society newsletter provides current information and describes what other sufferers have found helpful.

However all the information can be a bit confusing. You will not find straightforward answers; for example, you may have noticed that this book talks about 'pros and cons' of treatments and 'chances' of success. Without proper research, statements of fact by doctors and alternative practitioners may in reality merely be a matter of opinion. There is nothing wrong with opinions as such – after all, practitioners are trying to help women with endometriosis and what they are suggesting may well be worth trying – but it does mean you will come across conflicting views about the best approach. You may also come across doctors whose knowledge is simply out of date. If you investigate all the alternatives you will feel happier about the final decision.

Making decisions
Having endometriosis involves one decision after another, although at some stages you may not be given any options. You may find decision-making is straightforward, or you may feel

angry and rushed without the necessary information or time to think about it.

> The specialist recognised endometriosis and recommended I have a hysterectomy, which I decided to have.

> The amount of time a patient gets in the NHS outpatients is totally inadequate for the patient. The communication was terse, information limited, information exchange inadequate. Yet these are big decisions that need talking over.

Most people's decision-making is based on a mixture of thoughts and feelings. The best option is usually clear in simple decisions, and being wrong may not matter, but sufferers of endometriosis are often faced with complicated choices, for example about treatment or becoming pregnant.

Being more systematic in making difficult decisions can help you feel more confident and avoid later surprises or regrets. The accompanying box gives an outline of one way you may approach a decision. Although it looks very logical it does not exclude feelings you may have – these may seem irrational, but are none the less important.

QUICK GUIDE TO MAKING DECISIONS

Write down answers to the following in detail or talk them over with a friend.
- What is the problem?
- Is it important enough to spend time thinking about it?
- If yes, seek more information and help, e.g. from doctors, family and friends, support group, for the next steps.
- What are your alternatives? Write each alternative on a separate sheet of paper.
  What is likely to happen in each case?
  What are the immediately advantages and disadvantages?
  What are the long-term advantages and disadvantages?
- How do you *feel* about each alternative and any risks you might have to take? (Don't discount these feelings.)

- Can you try any of them out and change your mind?
  Are you prepared to accept the consequences of those you
  cannot reverse?

If you are faced with an important decision, it will help to
explore your options – and remember that doing nothing and
waiting to see what happens is also one of these options. This
chapter suggests many ways of getting further information and
discussing the problem with women who have had similar
experiences. Your decision may involve other people – your
partner for example – and you will need to get their reactions.
Do you know what their feelings are? Are you making any
assumptions about them?

Once you have worked out your options assess the chances of
success in each case, e.g. chances of conception with IVF, (page
100), chances of recurrence if ovaries remain (page 61). Then
think of the advantages and disadvantages in the immediate and
long-term. For example, danazol is likely to stop the pain but
you may get side effects (at which point you could try evening
primrose oil to combat them, or stop taking danazol). Buserelin
may help you get pregnant in the longer term but it is not the
answer if you have cysts. Surgery is a better alternative for cysts
but it is unpleasant initially and you will need time to recuperate.
Or think about an alternative approach; acupuncture could stop
pain and make you feel more positive, but you may need to find a
good practitioner and be able to pay.

You will obviously have feelings about each choice, but
sometimes the real reasons you do or don't like a particular
option can be difficult to pinpoint. You may think it is silly to
feel a particular way.

When I had both ovaries removed I thought I would age very
quickly.

You shouldn't look upon these emotions as silly, though. 'Silly'
feelings are real and part of examining all the options. Your
commitment to a sensible decision may be sapped, undermined,
by the feelings underneath – they are therefore not silly, but
important, and have to be faced up to and sorted out. It may

require a bit of careful thought and honesty with yourself, but if you let the feelings out then you can check your worries. You need to take into account your personal hopes and fears. If you dearly wish to conceive, you will probably opt for the treatment most likely to help, even if it may require a lot of effort. If you want to control pain, your choice may be different. Other priorities may be to maintain a good relationship with your partner, to feel good about yourself, to carry on with work or to avoid taking drugs all the time. You may have short-term goals as well, such as being fit to go on the holiday of a lifetime, not having surgery during exams, feeling fit for an interview, etc.

Your priorities may not be the same as your doctor's, so it is worth discussing with him or her what you want any treatment to achieve. Your doctor may put your physical health before other things which you see as equally important, e.g. feeling sexually attractive, the need to take account of domestic arrangements. Research has shown that patients are less likely to choose surgery than doctors are to suggest it. Talking to your doctor is a chance for concerns to be expressed before the final decision. This advice may seem rather irrelevant if your doctor is not actually offering you a choice. However, it is your health at stake, so you can ask for time to consider the matter and you do have the power to say no. You may be afraid of offending the doctor, but to do so is better than the shock of discovering you have not understood what is being suggested and of feeling the decision has been made for you.

She recommended hysterectomy and finally sterilised me, without proper counselling and advice, and caused me great grief and sorrow when I realised I could not have another child.

Getting in touch with others

My family and friends have been very helpful and supportive since my endometriosis was diagnosed but there has still been that isolated feeling of 'no one understands'. Now I know that lots of women understand – only too well!

I felt so elated because at last I could mention endometriosis and the whole group 'tuned in' and gave their experiences. We had a really good group therapy session. The leaflet read like a diary of my thoughts, feelings and fears.

Self help groups give you the opportunity to share your feelings with other people who know what it is like to have endometriosis. They can help you feel less isolated, and you may also feel better about talking to your doctor ('I didn't know anything about endometriosis so I didn't even know what questions to ask'). Some self-help groups teach new skills, such as pelvic-floor exercises and relaxation techniques, or simply provide a social night out and a way of making new friends. Certain sessions may be open to partners and husbands, giving them a chance to learn about endometriosis and to share their feelings.

Participating in or running a group can do wonders for feelings of helplessness and anger. It allows women to feel that at last they have found a way of fighting the disease by helping themselves and others.

The Endometriosis Society produces regular newsletters and provides a telephone helpline and a network of self-help groups throughout the UK. The National Fertility Association and the Hysterectomy Support Network are amongst other organisations who provide support (see useful addresses).

Depending on your technical skills and access to a computer with a modem, you can also get in touch with others through various discussion groups on the Internet (see page 170). For example, WITSENDO is an Internet group dedicated to endometriosis which some women have found very helpful:

It is now nine months since I was diagnosed, and I have become reconciled to living with a chronic disease and finding ways of overcoming it through the support of the women and men, doctors, researchers and patients who contribute to WITSENDO.

At first I just 'lurked' – listening to the messages but not making any contribution. On most e-mail lists, only about one tenth of subscribers actually contribute messages. It is quite OK to 'eavesdrop' and not to speak if you don't want to. Finally I plucked up courage and sent a first message giving my brief history and asking for information. It came flooding back.

I cannot recommend WITSENDO too strongly – even if all you want to do is tell someone who will understand how much pain you're in, or how much it upsets you that your partner tries to ignore your condition – WITSENDO is always there. Messages are posted by the moderator once a day normally, so although the response from other endo sufferers is not instant, when it comes it is quite overwhelming. They know how you feel, and they will joke, or offer advice or their own experience, or just rail along with you against the injustice of it all. But one final note or caution – don't take any decision on the basis of one message on WITSENDO. There is a wide spectrum of views and on a couple of occasions some rather off-the-wall advice has been given. When that happens, there is usually a cascade of other messages giving other points of view – and with experience you will know what weight you should give the views of different contributors. After all, on the Internet everyone is entitled to their view.

Other sources of support

People often tell horror stories about their doctors. (Your doctor probably feels the same way about builders or plumbers!) However many women have found their GP, gynaecologist or nurses very supportive. This is not to excuse those in medicine or nursing who have caused a lot of unnecessary grief or misunderstanding, but any profession is a mixture of people, and support and understanding will be available from somewhere.

Nursing staff were very kind and held my hand while I cried it all out of my system.

My husband and I would have given up more than once, but my gynaecologist does not give up easily and we are grateful to him for getting us this far.

It was fully explained to me by my own GP, who has been a tower of strength throughout the entire time.

Someone, somewhere understands and cares. Don't give up until you've exhausted every possibility that is available to you.

If you are unhappy with your GP or gynaecologist, then you can change your GP and perhaps be referred elsewhere (see page 29). However it may be that a doctor – any doctor – is simply not in a position to provide the emotional support you need, in which case you may need to become a member of a self-help group instead or consider other possibilities such as counselling, co-counselling or group therapy. They may sound a bit trendy, but sufferers have found them helpful.

A good counsellor can help you explore your emotions, your relationships with others and your feelings about treatments or decisions you have to make, rather than tell you what to do. A psychotherapist can help you think at a deeper level by looking at damaging experiences in early life and ways in which you have adopted negative emotional or behavioural patterns to cope, which may no longer be helpful now and may be contributing to your problems or to the endometriosis itself.

Counselling or therapy helps you change in positive ways. You may be afraid of exposing feelings you would rather not admit even to yourself. No one will force you to talk about them, but people often find a weight lifts when they reach a stage where they feel able to. You may also feel that going to someone for psychological help for endometriosis means admitting 'that it's all in your head'. You are certainly not declaring yourself mentally ill by seeking help: instead you are recognising that endometriosis is causing emotional problems which you can't resolve on your own and that going for help is a way of restoring your well-being.

Your GP or consultant may be able to refer you locally, although counselling and psychotherapy are limited on the NHS. Several voluntary organisations offer counselling services, but you will need to find out what is available in your area. Try contacting the British Association for Counselling or your local branch of MIND (the Mental Health Association) or the Samaritans for advice about local services or lists of counsellors. The Westminster Pastoral Association will put you in touch with a counsellor who can take account of your spiritual needs, if you wish. Relate (formerly known as the Marriage Guidance Council) or the Child Guidance Service (may be called the Child and Family Consultation Service) provide help where problems have become focused on the area of family relationships (look them up in the phone book). Women's Therapy Centres are another possible source of help. You will often have to see a counsellor privately, which can be expensive although some organisations operate a sliding scale of charges, so it is worth asking before you decide you can't afford it.

Co-counselling is a technique in which you are paired with someone and take it in turns to focus on the other's problems, meeting on a regular basis and sticking to certain guidelines. It has the advantage of being cheap and flexible, but you may find you need the skills and insight of a trained counsellor, or that you feel too needy to be able to offer much to someone else.

As for group therapy, there are innumerable varieties. You can find out what might suit you from *A Complete Guide to Therapy* (see recommended reading). The organisations mentioned above and women's health centres may know of suitable groups in your area.

I have found group therapy very effective in helping with emotional aspects of being ill and in redirecting energies wasted in worrying.

9
GETTING TO GRIPS WITH PAIN

by Lesley Misrahi

For most sufferers, endometriosis *is* pain. You know you've got the disease or that it has returned because you recognise the pain. Many women might not mind being riddled with endometriosis if it didn't affect fertility and cause pain. Some doctors have gone so far as to suggest that, since treatment for endometriosis is long, often with unpleasant side effects, and surgery can result in scarring, they should treat the pain rather than the endometriosis. However, it is also true that many of the treatment options discussed in Chapters 3 and 4 have given sufferers 'time out' from pain, sometimes lasting years.

This chapter dwells on pain in order to illustrate the ways in which endometriosis sufferers have tried to change their lives, deal with their pain and look towards a brighter future.

> Since stopping the tablets I still feel very well. It might be because I am free of monthly pain for the first time in my life and that does the trick. It is an indescribable feeling.

> I feel better now than I have done for 20 years and it is so good to be able to plan things ahead.

ENDOMETRIOSIS AND PAIN

Women with endometriosis report many types of pain, but ironically endometriosis is not necessarily painful. Sufferers can have severe endometriosis and no painful symptoms (see Chapter 2). However, there is some evidence that women with endometriosis and/or adhesions report painful periods (dysmenorrhoea), deep pain during sex (dyspareunia), pain after sex and persistent pain during the cycle more often than women without the disease and that endometriosis is more likely to be found amongst women complaining of severe painful periods than those with milder dysmenorrhoea.

The way in which endometriosis causes pain is not well understood. As discussed in Chapter 2, it appears that younger, *deeper* patches of endometriosis of various colours are associated with painful symptoms. Pain may be felt when nerve endings are stimulated by irritating substances released either by active endometriosis or the inflammation it causes. Alternatively, pain may result from actual tissue damage caused by infiltrating endometriosis or by inflammation and scarring.

The peritoneum, where endometriosis usually deposits, is very sensitive so inflammation develops easily as the body tries to heal the area. High levels of chemicals such as prostaglandins have been found in the peritoneal fluid of endometriosis sufferers and these can aggravate nerve endings and cause painful muscle spasms. Sensitive areas may also produce mid-cycle pain if irritated by fluids normally released from the ovary during ovulation. The growth of 'chocolate' cysts on the ovary is usually painless but if they rupture and spill their contents onto the peritoneum, they will set off an intense inflammatory reaction causing a severe acute attack of pain.

Painful sex may be explained by the penis stretching endometriosis or adhesions on the uterosacral ligaments supporting the uterus. In some cases, the penis may be bumping an ovary trapped by adhesions behind the uterus (normally the ovaries would be free to slide to one side).

Adhesions can cause pain after the endometriosis has gone because internal organs are stuck together in uncomfortable positions. This may account for dragging sensations, painful bowel movements, painful sex and sharp pains in pregnancy or due to sudden movement when adhesions are pulled.

However, doctors do not really know how endometriosis causes pain, or why the pain is so severe in some sufferers, yet doesn't appear in others. The fact that it is difficult to measure hampers research and can make it hard to convince your doctor

94% suffer from period pain, severe for 66%.

Cramps extend down my legs to my knees and sometimes to my ankles. I am in extreme pain from my waist to my toes.

77% have ovulation pain, severe for 30%.

A DULL ACHING NAGGING PAIN ON RIGHT SIDE AT OVULATION, GOING DOWN INTO MY VAGINA

57% experience pain at any time of the month.

A definite bruising feeling from one hip bone to the other. On the days without pain the whole area feels as if I had been kicked.

55% have a painful sexual intercourse. 3% said this meant they couldn't try for a baby.

Sharp pain on deep penetration. Much worse in certain positions.

48% suffer painful defaecation.

6-7 days before onset of periods pain on opening bowels

37% get back pain during periods. 42% have it most of the time.

BACK-PAIN, SOMETIMES DURING PERIODS OR AT OVULATION, WITH PAIN IN THE RIGHT LEG

32% are kept awake by pain.

I found I could not sleep on my back or sides so I used to 'sit-up' with the aid of many pillows

26% found urination caused pain.

SEVERE PAINS IN THE FRONT PASSAGE PAINFUL TO START URINATION & MAINTAIN A FLOW OF URINE

Common pains reported by sufferers in the Endometriosis Society Survey.

about the extent of your pain, especially when it isn't related to the amount of endometriosis.

> The surgeon's visual inspection indicates that it's not severe. However, I find the pain crippling, and totally inhibiting to my usual lifestyle.

> My GP was helpful but both he and the consultant took a long time to take account of the terrible pain it caused.

If a pain meter could give an instant reading, perhaps your doctor would be more helpful. Try using the pain chart overleaf to record your pain. Although it will be subjective, it may help your doctor understand what you are going through. Or use it to

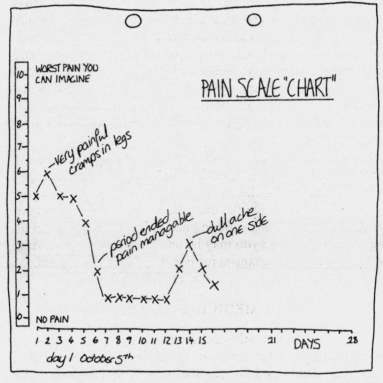

Pain Scale.

see how well some of the pain-relief methods described in this chapter work for you.

HOW PAIN RELIEF WORKS

Put simply, pain is a message from a part of your body which is suffering real or potential damage, telling your brain to do something about it. Pain relief interrupts the transmission of the pain message at different points along its path. Research suggests that dull aches travel by one route into the brain, while sharp stabbing pains pass along another – which explains why some pain-relief methods affect one type of sensation while leaving the other untouched.

Aspirin and related drugs block the production of prostaglandins, reducing any inflammation and interfering with the formation of pain messages at nerve endings. Narcotic drugs block pain messages at critical sites in the spinal cord and brain. One way they do this is by imitating endorphins, chemicals which are the body's natural painkillers. Both narcotics and endorphins can attach to receptors in the brain and spinal cord producing a painkilling effect and a feeling of well-being. Endorphins can be stimulated by sustained exercise such as running and aerobics, and by using techniques such as acupuncture and shiatsu to treat pain.

The way pain is perceived once it reaches the brain depends on attitudes, expectations, thoughts and feelings. For example, research suggests that distracting people can reduce their pain by as much as a third. On the other hand, if you're expecting to hurt, or perhaps if the suffering actually rescues you from an unpleasant situation, you may be unconsciously concentrating on the pain. The mechanism for this is not well understood.

THE MEDICINE CABINET

Over-the-counter medicines

Several mild painkillers are available at the pharmacist. Aspirin reduces any fever and inflammation, as well as killing pain, but it can cause stomach irritation and bleeding. These side effects can be reduced by taking it with food or milk, using soluble tablets, or trying another drug in the salicylate family (e.g. benorylate, salicylamide although you may need a prescription for this). Ibuprofen is another popular anti-inflammatory and mild painkiller, but it can also irritate the stomach lining. Paracetamol is a good alternative painkiller if you cannot tolerate these side effects, but it does not reduce inflammation.

You will find many brands of aspirin or paracetamol or both. There is no evidence that combinations of these drugs are more effective and it is often an expensive way of taking them. You may be surprised to find caffeine included in some preparations. It may make the painkiller more effective, but it is a stimulant and can keep you awake at night. Read the label to make sure what any compound contains – and don't take even mild painkillers for more than ten consecutive days without medical advice. Do discuss over-the-counter drugs with your GP because they can interact with other medicines.

Anti-spasmodic drugs in the hyoscine family can relieve period pain. Endometriosis sufferers have found Feminax, which includes this type of drug, a useful standby so it is worth a try if you can tolerate all its ingredients (salicylamide, paracetamol, codeine, hyoscine hydrobromide and caffeine). Read the label for precautions, because anti-spasmodics can cause nausea and drowsiness.

If you want a stronger painkiller, you can buy many preparations containing codeine, but you should be careful about relying on them for regular use since codeine belongs to the narcotic family (see below). Codeine often causes constipation, which might cause further discomfort, especially if your endometriosis affects your bowel.

If over-the-counter medicines don't help, or give you stomach upsets or constipation, your GP may be able to prescribe a stronger drug or one with fewer side effects.

Prescribed painkillers

Several trials have been done comparing aspirin with prescribed anti-inflammatory drugs such as indomethacin, tolfenamic acid and naproxen sodium (Synflex) to see whether they helped pain in women with endometriosis more than taking a placebo (see page 73). Tolfenamic acid and naproxen sodium reduced painful periods more effectively than aspirin or indomethacin which were no more effective than a placebo. Your GP will be able to prescribe Synflex but tolfenamic acid is not available in the UK. However, many sufferers have found the related compound, mefenamic acid (Ponstan), to be helpful. These drugs belong to the family know as non-steroidal anti-inflammatories (NSAIDS). NSAIDs can irritate the stomach lining unless you take them with food or drink of milk and cannot be used long term.

Your GP may also suggest stronger drugs related to codeine such as dihydrocodeine (DF 118) or dextromoramide, although they can also produce constipation and shouldn't be used daily because of the risk of dependence. A similar drug, dextropropoxyphene, is included with paracetamol in co-proxamol (Distalgesic).

Equagesic is sometimes prescribed for pain. It includes aspirin and ethoheptazine citrate, another mild pain-reliever, and meprobamate, a tranquilliser that can cause addiction if used reguarly. Pentazocine (Fortral and in Fortagesic) may be recommended for moderate to severe pain since its strength lies between that of codeine and morphine. However, it tends to cause nausea and vomiting. It is more effective when injected, but can cause hallucinations, and regular injection has resulted in dependence.

Your doctor will probably be unwilling to prescribe something stronger for any length of time because many moderate and severe painkillers are narcotics, well-known for their tendency to cause physiological addiction (when the body develops a physical need for the drug) and psychological dependence (when people have a craving and feel they can't cope without it) if used regularly. They may also produce tolerance, when an increasing dose is needed to produce the same effect.

If you suffer from severe pain, you may remember the painkilling effects of morphine or pethidine used after surgery and wish your doctor could prescribe something similar. However, the more effective a drug is for killing pain, the more likely it is to cause side effects or addiction. Morphine and related narcotics are not suitable for regular use because patients can become dependent after two to four weeks, even on low doses, and severe withdrawal symptoms can occur if treatment stops.

Tranquillisers, sleeping pills, anti-depressants or anti-convulsants can also be prescribed for chronic pain. Research trials on anti-depressants such as Amitriptyline or anti-convulsants such as Mexiletine have shown they are helpful for chronic pain, although this research wasn't done on endometriosis sufferers. Taking these drugs does not mean you are mentally ill or that your endometriosis is psychosomatic: emotional states contribute to how we experience pain, so these drugs can help pain temporarily by reducing anxiety or depression, or encouraging sleep. However, long-term use of drugs such as Valium or Mogadon can reduce your pain tolerance, interfere with sleep and cause depression. Some sleeping pills and painkillers combine to produce more rather than less pain if taken together, though long-term use of drugs such as Valium, Ativan and Mogadon can lead to addiction.

Relying on painkillers can be a very frustrating process of juggling the benefits and side effects of different drugs, and there are no miracles. If you are being prescribed a painkiller which you feel isn't helping enough, talk to your doctor. You might gain relief from trying a different type of painkiller (e.g. an anti-inflammatory such as Ponstan or Synflex, or codeine-type drugs such as Distalgesic or DF 118 for the worst days). Equally, if the painkilling effect is good but you have bad side effects, another drug could be more suitable.

If you use prescribed painkillers regularly, you may be alarmed to read about the side effects and dangers mentioned above. If the drug has not caused problems, you are probably one of the majority for whom it is all right. You can get further information from the British Medical Association's *Guide to Medicines and Drugs* or the *British National Formulary* (see recommended reading), but talk to your doctor if you are worried. If you are taking a drug regularly which may be addictive, try not taking it for a bit. If symptoms such as pains, cravings, nervousness, etc., develop, start taking the drug again and consult your doctor immediately for advice and support in withdrawing from it slowly. This chapter suggests several alternative ways of controlling pain, so you will not be left stranded.

DLPA: a nutritional painkiller

DLPA is a mixture of two forms (known as *D-* and *L-*) of phenylalanine, an amino-acid constituent of food proteins. It has been found to reduce pain when taken regularly, it is thought, by blocking enzymes which destroy endorphins, the body's own painkillers. Endometriosis sufferers have found DLPA helpful, sometimes for specific components of their pain.

> I can't tell you how glad I am that a friend passed on details of the DLPA treatment. My chronic back pain has not responded to steroid injections, morphine or pethidine drugs. (I am unable to take codeine or aspirin). Already, the general level of pain is lowered and I can now 'pace myself' each day without being overwhelmed by pain. This is the best news in three dreadful years.

Tablets are taken for several weeks, rather than when you are in pain. The initial dose of 375 mg twice daily is gradually increased to 2 x 375 mg three times a day. Once this dose is reached, pain relief should start within a few days and persist for two to three weeks after the end of treatment.

DLPA is non-addictive and you don't have to take longer and larger doses for the same effect. A few sufferers have reported severe indigestion as a side effect. DLPA should not be used in pregnancy, and those with high blood pressure should take it after meals.

DLPA can be used with any existing treatment, including aspirin or anti-flammatory drugs. Vitamins B6 and C appear to make DLPA more effective if they are taken at the same time. If you can't get DLPA locally, the Endometriosis Society may be able to advise you.

Alternative remedies

Endometriosis sufferers report that various supplements help pain, e.g. selenium, evening primrose oil and calcium (see Chapter 5). Several home remedies are recommended, but you should consult a medical herbalist or homoeopath for more specific advice.

- A pinch of powdered ginger or a few shreds of root ginger in a cup of boiling water sipped at regular intervals (sweeten with honey if desired) relieves spasms and improves circulation.
- One teaspoon of essence of peppermint, eight teaspoons of oil of orange, eight teaspoons of oil of ginger, in a pint of water. One tablespoon to be taken in a glass of hot water for period pain.
- Thyme tea is also advocated for gynaecological pain.
- Angelica root is a traditional remedy from China, boiled as a kind of soup and taken throughout the cycle.

PHYSICAL TREATMENTS FOR PAIN

Transcutaneous electrical nerve stimulation

Transcutaneous electrical nerve stimulation (TENS) is based on the idea that nerves can be stimulated to prevent pain messages from the damaged site reaching the brain. A small battery-operated device generates a series of pulses which stimulate nerves via two electrodes stuck on the skin with conducting paste. The process is painless and studies have shown that 65–95 per cent of patients with a variety of conditions benefit in the short term, with 30–50 per cent of people still experiencing relief months later. A study of women with pelvic pain, using a similar method for one hour daily for one and a half months, showed 30–50 per cent relief after a week and 60–80 per cent after 20 treatments.

TENS appears to work best for persistent pain. Side effects are minimal – sometimes a slight rash from the electrode paste – although it should not be used if you are pregnant or have a pacemaker (see manufacturer's instructions). Your GP may be able to refer you to your local physiotherapy department for advice and a possible free loan or you may want to buy one. Some medical equipment suppliers (see Yellow Pages and useful addresses) will allow sale or return, or refund part of the purchase price if it does not work for you. Some hospital pain clinics can lend you one to see if it works.

Acupuncture

The ancient Chinese art of acupuncture is thought to work in a similar way to TENS; it is said to restore energy flows in the body, dispersing pain and allowing healing. Diagnosis before acupuncture treatment is made by feeling pulses in different parts of the body. Treatment then involves stimulating specific points with needles for varying lengths of time. Acupuncture needles are very fine, and skilled insertion is almost painless. The needles may then be rotated or electrically stimulated, or the herb moxa may be burnt over the sites (moxibustion).

In a consumer survey in *Which?* magazine (October 1986), nearly a quarter of 446 people who had used acupuncture for chronic pain said they were cured, almost another half reported improvement and 60 per cent said they would definitely use it again and recommend it to others. Some endometriosis sufferers have found it beneficial; others have not. As with many treatments (including surgery!) you may suffer more before you get better, so don't give up too soon.

For a list of qualified practitioners who will exercise proper safeguards against the spread of disease by needles, write to the Council for Acupuncture (see useful addresses). Doctors who use acupuncture belong to the British Medical Acupuncture Society.

Forms of therapeutic massage

There are several specialist forms of massage, well known for relaxing the body and relieving pain.

Acupressure is a Chinese first-aid technique which uses finger-pressure to stimulate acupuncture points. It was developed into shiatsu by the Japanese. Both have the merit that it is possible to learn to do them yourself, or you can ask a friend to learn. A qualified practitioner will be able to ascertain what pressure points are appropriate to you; for example, try rubbing the point in the hollow just below your knee for period pain – feel around till you find a place that is slightly tender and then rub with the thumb for about 10 minutes.

Reflexology relies on stimulating points on the feet which correspond with the body's organs.

Aromatherapy is a form of massage using essential oils which are believed to have therapeutic properties (see Chapter 5). Oils which promote relaxation (e.g. lavender) or specifically for pain (e.g. jasmine) may be helpful (see recommended reading or consult an aromatherapist).

Contact community centres, adult education departments, yoga teachers, health farms, gyms and health clubs to find out about local practitioners, courses and workshops.

Heat and cold

Many people find a warm bath, shower, sauna or using a hot-water bottle or heating pad helps pain, and endometriosis sufferers are no exception. And cold is said to be even more effective than heat. Rub a cold object (e.g. a hot-water bottle filled with crushed ice or cold compress gel pack available from chemists) over the painful site. Keep it moving all the time. As soon as your skin feels numb, stop treatment and start moving that part of the body again. It should feel better.

Exercises for pelvic pain

Just as movement is best for a leg cramp, so your pelvic muscles need to be gently exercised rather than being allowed to carry on contracting spasmodically. If possible try the following, rather than curling up in bed.

- Lie on your back with your feet propped up against a wall. Stay there for five to ten minutes.
- Lie on your back on the floor or bed and, keeping one leg still, bring the other one up towards your chin, bending the knee. Hold it there with your hands for a few minutes, then try the other leg.
- Kneel on the floor. Rest your forearms so your elbows are on the floor in front of you, with your head between your arms. Rock gently backwards and forwards with your head alternately between your arms and above your hands.

THE VICIOUS CIRCLE

What do you feel when you are in pain? Do you anticipate more pain? Worry about needing surgery? Remember you have got endometriosis or that you are infertie? Feel angry about your plans being spoilt? Feel guilty about your partner or children having to put up with you? Feel it is unfair and people don't understand what you are going through?

If I am emotionally unhappy, the pain worsens.

At the moment I know that although my chances of pregnancy are small, they would be much better if I could only get rid of the pain for a while. I could then forget my non-pregnant state, relax more and give myself a better chance of conceiving.

The way you feel about your pain can have a considerable effect on its intensity. Pain can be made better or worse by how you respond to it, and yet depression and anxiety are a natural response to being debilitated. You can end up in a vicious circle. This doesn't mean it is your fault if you are in terrible pain or feeling angry or demoralised by it: but it does mean that you can harness the most potent pain-control agent there is – your mind. This may seem unlikely, but it is effective.

What do you do when you are in pain? Do you rub the sore place? Cry? Tell other people and ask them to help? Avoid doing anything that makes it hurt? Get some rest? Take medicine? Go to the doctor? These can be good strategies for short-term pain relief because they give the body a chance to heal itself. But if the pain gets no better or keeps coming back, you need, a different approach to prevent you from becoming an invalid, unable to lead a normal life.

Many endometriosis sufferers (and other people who suffer from chronic pain) have found that a change in lifestyle can help to prevent pain occurring, and minimises it when it does. They have learnt to manage their pain by making changes in their daily routine and thinking more positively. Many people find this easier to do if they have support, either from their family, a self-help group or even professional advice from a NHS pain clinic (ask your GP if there is one in your area). The clinic will devise a regime of pain-control techniques and teach you ways out of the vicious circle of feelings and pain. You can try developing your own programme using the following sections.

A PAIN-CONTROL PROGRAMME

Being positive and wholehearted

You can make your life more comfortable and take steps to deal with the pain, but you will have to face the pain and decide to do something positive. This involves accepting that there is no instant cure for your distress, but that you can take many different steps to help yourself.

Most thoughts about pain are negative, which can lead to more anxiety and more pain. If you think you can't cope, you probably won't. But how do you stop understandable feelings of panic?

Research on women due to have gynaecological surgery has shown that a simple exercise where they were asked to list their fears and then revise them more positively helped women feel better about the operation, and they needed fewer painkillers afterwards. So, prior to your next bout of pain, think of things to say to yourself to counteract the inevitable negative feelings. Those based on your previous experience are probably best.

This is killing me.	This isn't going to kill me and if I can get through the next hour, it will ease off a bit.
It is getting worse.	It will get better if I relax.
Painkillers make me feel ill and don't help.	Maybe I can try DLPA or the recommended exercises.

It can be very difficult to give up negative ways of coping if you are confusing your emotional needs with your pain. For example, you may feel people only care about you when you are not well or only ask you how you are feeling when you are in pain. You may only allow yourself to rest when you are in pain, or that may be the only time you ask other people to take over some of your commitments.

Everyone needs to feel cared for whether or not they are in pain. You and your family may have got into the habit of forgetting about your needs unless you are in pain. Try asking your partner or children to get their own meals more often, not just when you are ill. Give yourself a break before the pain gets worse, not when you've collapsed. Ask your partner for love, concern and help when you need it, not just when you are in pain and your partner feels obliged to give it. Do something special together when you're feeling better, so you feel you are giving something in return and not just 'a moaning old ratbag at 27'.

Keeping your mind active

Keep busy. Try to maintain your daily activities as far as possible, especially those you enjoy. It has been found that those who go to bed with period pains are likely to suffer more than those who try to do things to take their minds off their pain. Reading a book, watching TV, talking to friends are activities more likely to be helpful. At the height of the spasms even singing a song can help distract you from the intensity of the pain.

> When the pain is bad, I have to give myself a serious mental talk i.e. if people can fight cancer, why can't I fight this?

This does not mean being stoical and keeping going until you collapse. Endometriosis sufferers need to be kind to themselves by assessing their needs and asking others to help at the right time, instead of just when they are suffering. General support can help you fight the pain when it is bad.

Keeping your body active

Many people cope with chronic pain by becoming increasingly inactive. This can make matters worse since whole groups of muscles can remain virtually unused. Loss of tone in the back and abdominal muscles can then lead to back injuries and strains, causing further painful problems.

> I had really awful back pains – usual endometriosis-type pain, but much worse. I was nearly screaming with pain when I tottered into the surgery. It turned out to be lumbago; nothing to do with endometriosis at all.

Exercise prevents these problems, but if you are going to do it regularly, it has to be enjoyable. What about the following? If you find walking, stretching or vibration painful, choose something gentle.

- Aerobics, running and cycling are often recommended for getting you fit and stimulating the flow of endorphins (the body's natural painkillers). Choose this sort of exercise if you don't have too much of a pain-barrier to overcome.
- Walk at your own pace, somewhere you enjoy. Some people recommended getting a dog.
- Yoga is a complete therapy, as well as exercise. Try it if stretching is not too painful. There may be teachers locally.
- Swimming exercises the whole body. The water is supportive, preventing some of the dragging pain you may get when standing or walking. Try the exercises opposite.
- Dancing needn't be at a disco. You can put on your favourite record and be as mild or wild as you like in your own home.
- Alexander technique and Feldenkreiss method are both designed to reduce pain in your daily life by improving posture and muscle tone. There may be classes locally.

Keeping your pelvic-floor muscles in good condition (see Chapter 1) helps avoid some of the painful problems caused by surgery, lack of oestrogen, childbirth and constipation.

Learning to relax

For the first time in my life I feel in control. Now that I have the ability to relax I get so much more out of life and don't spend half my time worrying about what may or may not ever happen.

Relaxation is an invaluable skill for everyone, but it is especially helpful if you suffer from chronic pain. You don't have to find a dark room and half an hour a day where you are uninterrupted, although they will help.

You can learn breathing and muscle tensing and relaxing exercises which you can do anywhere, even stopped at traffic lights in the car, but you will need to spend more time on relaxation if you are going to help chronic pain. You can buy relaxation and pain-control tapes, or there may be relaxation classes locally. Yoga and autogenic training are therapies which teach relaxation.

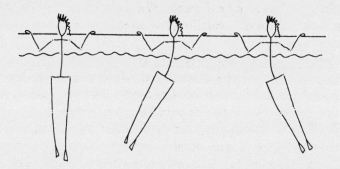

Waist Swing.

Hold onto the rail. Relax with your legs straight and together. Gently swing your body and legs from the waist down, first to one side, then the other. Keep your upper body and shoulders still. Repeat five times each side and increase to 20.

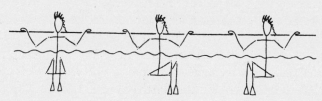

Waist twist.

Hold onto the rail. Draw your knees up to your chest. Holding this position with your knees pressed together, twist as far as you can to the right. Hold for four or five seconds. Return to middle and then repeat movement to the left. Return to the middle and repeat exercise. Complete sequence five times and increase to 20 times.

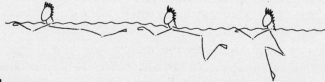

Curl-ups

Hold onto the rail, with arms bent and legs stretched out behind you. Grip your legs together and slowly bend your knees up towards your chest. Hold for four or five seconds. Relax. Repeat exercise. Start with five and increase to 20 times.

There are no special clothes or equipment for autogenic training. The therapist guides the group through a set of exercises which warms your limbs, steadies your heartbeat and calms your breathing. After four weeks there was a marvellous lifting of anxiety. I cheered up tremendously. My aches and pains diminished as my muscles unknotted. I was amazed to find that everyday things which had caused me problems were really quite easy. There have been ups and downs since but perhaps life doesn't get me in the same way. Nothing succeeds like success and if you've had even a week of feeling calm and healthy, you know it can happen again and it will.

This method of relaxation has helped me live with the complaint by reducing pain and releasing additional energy to take up activities to promote my well-being – dancing and painting.

The key to relaxation is breathing. Most of us breathe by inflating the upper parts of our chests. When in distress we breathe more and more shallowly. To relax, you need to take deep, slow breaths, by lowering your diaphragm, rather than raising your ribcage. If you practise this, just taking a few deep breaths will help you to calm down when you feel bad.

Sit comfortably or lie on your back, close your eyes and breathe deeply and slowly. Become aware of each part of your body in turn, beginning with your feet and moving upwards to your head. If a part of your body feels tense consciously relax it. (It helps some people to tense up each group of muscles and then allow them to relax.) Pay special attention to the muscles of your neck, shoulders and face. Now imagine yourself in a pleasant natural setting and concentrate on the details of this special place while continuing to breathe deeply and easily. After some minutes of relaxation, you can gradually let yourself return to your everyday life and open your eyes.

Visualisation

Just as emotional difficulties can promote endometriosis, (see Chapter 8) your mind can also help to make you well. Visualisation seeks to harness your powers of imagination to heal your body. It involves picturing to yourself, in a symbolic way, the processes needed for your life to improve, while you are deeply relaxed. The way you imagine things can be as silly as you like – they only need to have meaning for you and to express as powerfully as possible the goal you are trying to achieve.

Try adding to your relaxation the following exercise to improve your condition: After you have reached a relaxed state and are feeling comfortable, imagine the endometriosis cells in your body. See them weak and confused because they are in the wrong place. Now imagine the purposeful army of white blood cells, your body's natural defenders, flooding in as the blood flow round your pelvis improves. They destroy and dispose of the unwanted cells, tidying up scar tissue and soothing inflammation. Imagine all your organs pink and healthy and your hormones balanced. See yourself healthy and full of energy, getting what you want out of life. After about 10 minutes, gradually allow yourself to return to normal, having assured yourself that you are going to feel better.

Practised regularly at least once a day, this technique can help. It's even helped 'incurable' cancer. But your images should be convincing. If it looks like the endometriosis cells might win or you can't really imagine yourself happy and healthy, you need to consider whether your unconscious mind has reasons for keeping you ill. You can do this best by allowing yourself to fantasise about life without endometriosis as you are relaxing.

You can also use this technique specifically for pain (see box) or for other problems in your life.

VISUALISATION TECHNIQUES FOR PAIN

First relax using your favourite method. Then try one of the following.
- Imagine that your hand is very cold, so that it becomes numb. Now put your hand where the pain is and allow the numbness to soak through your skin to anaesthetise the pain.
- Visualise one of your hands as being your uterus. Concentrate on making the illusion as real as possible. Tense your

hand up into a fist and then let the muscles relax, allowing the uterine muscle to relax as well.

- Visualise your pain as an animal. Make it as real as possible. Now have a dialogue with it. Ask it why it is there, what its purpose is and what its message is. Ask what you must do to make it go away. Listen to it and do what it says.

Eating well

Everybody tells you to have a good diet if you want to keep well. Your local clinic or health education department (see under your district health authority in the phone book) will have leaflets on how to reduce fat intake while maintaining adequate protein and vitamin levels.

Pay particular attention to fibre intake – bowel symptoms are a huge problem with endometriosis sufferers. Fibre can aid constipation and level out fluctuations between diarrhoea and constipation. You don't need bran with everything (too much can make things worse at first), but eat plenty of whole grains, fruit and vegetables.

Try to control your intake of caffeine and alcohol as these can add to your body's physical reactions to stress and may exacerbate pain in the long run.

Enjoying sex again

Endometriosis can make sex hell for you, and not much fun for your partner. This seems to be a particular problem in heterosexual relationships, because penetration can produce sharp pains deep in the pelvis or leave women feeling 'as if I've been kicked' for some time afterwards. Other women find orgasm starts painful contractions, which may be worse during drug treatment if the uterine muscle becomes hypersensitive. Painful sex (dyspareunia) is one of the most difficult problems endometriosis sufferers and their partners have to face, but there are things you can do to help yourselves – and each other.

Painful sex is a shared problem which you need to talk about. You may be the one in pain, but your partner doesn't want to hurt you. You are both likely to feel angry and frustrated by the endometriosis, anxious about making love and worried that the problem will cause you to drift apart. Your expectations of each other may change, without either of you knowing what the other is feeling.

> He always used to say 'I love you' during sex. I didn't want him to say it any more (or even make love to me). How could he mean it when he knew it hurt me? When we talked I realised that he hadn't stopped loving me because of the endometriosis, and naturally still had sexual feelings, but hated the idea of hurting me. Together we found it was much better when I was on top; penetration wasn't as deep and I was more in control and able to move if I thought it was going to hurt.

Your partner may feel rejected, or that you don't enjoy sex any more, when the truth is that you don't enjoy the pain, rather than sex itself or being with your partner. You may fear your partner will leave you for a woman without endometriosis. You can only get each other's reassurance if you talk about your fears. Talking can also help you work out ways to continue sharing your sexuality.

Give yourselves more time and ask each other for encouragement and stimulation. Working together to make sure you are sexually aroused before penetration can help enormously – you become lubricated, your vagina elongates and the cervix moves higher up so there is less impact on it and other pelvic organs. You are less likely to contract the muscles at the vaginal entrance involuntarily (vaginismus). Vaginismus may develop if you have experienced a lot of pain. It can make penetration uncomfortable or even impossible, but often improves when you begin to feel more relaxed.

Working together to make sure your partner is aroused can help him feel less rejected – he will find it easier to be more caring if he feels less rejected – he will find it easier to be more caring if he feels you are encouarging his sexuality rather than trying to dampen it down. Remember there is no rush, and penetration isn't everything. It can be fun to delay it as long as possible, or rule out penetration for several weeks while you experiment with other ways of making love. This will help you regain confidence in each other and even rejuvenate your love-making. If penetration is still painful later on, then you will feel able to share your sexuality in different ways while you are getting treatment.

Several physical problems, apart from your endometriosis, may be contributing to your pain, and are worth checking. Lack of lubrication when you are sexually aroused may be due to lack of oestrogen because of drug treatment, breastfeeding, removal of your ovaries or the natural menopause. Try KY Jelly from the chemists as a lubricant, or rub a little vitamin E oil into your vagina. Your doctor may prescribe oestrogen creams or hormone replacement therapy if you are menopausal (see page 63). Pain in your vagina or vulva could be due to an infection of thrush, which is common during hormone treatment. Ask your doctor to check in case you need treatment.

You may have the added problem of infertility, and desperately what a baby. Your sex life may become governed by your menstrual cycle and the need for penetration; you can the get into a vicious circle where sex becomes too unhappy and painful. Consider talking to your doctor about artificial insemination (using your partner's sperm) to take the pressure off your sexual relationship while giving you a chance to conceive.

If you feel your relationship will not be helped by any of the above, then you (and your partner) may need outside support to help you sort out the difficulties that painful sex is causing. You may feel it would be too embarrassing to talk to someone else about your problems, but many people have been helped by seeing a counsellor. And counselling may be able to help sort out problems in your relationship which may be contributing to the pain.

Talking to someone can also help you if you are single and previous experiences of painful sex are preventing you from even wanting to start a new relationship. Try asking your GP to refer you, or contact the local branch of Relate (used to be called the Marriage Guidance Council) or Family Planning Association. Both Relate and the FPA are happy to help unmarried or gay women.

Good luck!

RECOMMENDED READING

Books on endometriosis
for women (and their doctors)

Ballweg M. and Deutsch S. (1988) *Overcoming Endometriosis*, Arlington
An American text written by members of the American Endometriosis Assocation.

Breitkopf L. J. and Bakoulis M.G. (1993) *Endometriosis: A Guide to One of the Most Common Causes of Period Pains and Infertility*, Thorsons
An American text by a doctor and colleague.

Hayman S. (1991) *Endometriosis*, Penguin
British text.

Henderson L., Riley R. and Wood R. (1991) *Explaining Endometriosis*, Allen & Unwin
Written by members of the Endometriosis Association of Victoria, Australia.

Lark S.M. (1993) *Fibroid tumours and Endometriosis*, Westchester Publishing Co
Written by an American doctor; useful range of exercises to help with pain management.

Lauersen N.H. (1988) *The endometriosis answer book: new hope/new help*, Ballantine
American text.

Older J. (1984) *Endometriosis*, Scribners
First American book.

Sachs J. (1991) *What Women can do about Chronic Endometriosis*, Dell Publishing
American text.

Third Side Press (1994) *Alternatives for Women with Endometriosis: a Guide by Women for Women*,
American text.

Weinstein (1987) *Living with Endometriosis*, Addison-Wesley
In-depth American book about coping with the disease.

Other Useful books

British Medical Association (1994) *New Guide to Medicines and Drugs*, Dorling Kindersley

British National Formulary (doctors' guide to drugs) published annually by the British Medical Association and the The Pharmaceutical Society of Great Britain.

Charles R. (1990) *Mind, Body and Immunity*, Cedar

Dennerstein L., Wood C. and Burroughs G. (1986) *Hysterectomy; How to Deal with the Physical and Emotional Aspects*, Oxford University Press

Dickson A. (1994) *A Woman in your Own Right*, Quartet

Gann, R. (1991) *The Health Care Consumer Guide*, Faber & Faber

Kovel J. (1978) *A Complete Guide to Therapy*, Penguin

Norwood R. (1994) *Why Me, Why This, Why Now*, Century

Pfeffer N. and Woollett A. (1983) *The Experience of Infertility*, Virago

Phillips A. and Rakusen J. (1991) *Our Bodies Ourselves*, Penguin

Rakusen J. (1987) *The Menopause: A Guide for all Ages* Purchase from: National Extension College, 18 Brooklands Avenue, Cambridge CB2 2EN.

Shapiro J. (1989) *Ourselves growing Older*, Fontana

Sheehy G. (1994) *The Silent Passage: Menopause*, Harper Collins

Trevelyan J. and Booth B. (1994) *Complementary Medicine for Nurses, Midwives and Health Visitors*, MacMillan

Westcott P. (1987) *Alternative Health Care for Women*, Thorsons

Winston R. (1994) *Infertility: A Sympathetic Approach*, Vermilion

Woodham A. (1995) *A Guide to Complementary Medicine and Therapies*, Health Education Authority

Worwood V. A. (1990) *The Fragrant Pharmacy*, Bantam
Specific guidance on aromatherapy for endometriosis.

Medical books and a sample of research papers for future reading

(1991) 'Endometriosis in the 1990s', *British Journal of Clinical Practice*, (45)3, Autumn, Symposium Supplement 72 (a series of articles)

(1992) 'Endometriosis', *British Journal of Obstetrics and Gynaecology*, Feb. 99 Supplement 7 (a series of articles)

(1992) 'Endometriosis: time for reappraisal', *Lancet*, Oct. 31, 340 (8827): 1073 (editoral)

Brosens I. and Donnez J. (1993) 'The Current State of Endometriosis and Management', *Proceedings of the 3rd World Congress*, Brussels, June 1992

Brosens I. (ed.) (1993) Endometriosis, *Baillière's Clinical Obstetrics and Gynaecology: International Practice and Research*, vol. 7, no. 4, Baillière Tindall

Brosens I. (ed) (1994) *Endometriosis: New Principles in Practice*, World Congress of Human Reproduction

Darrow S.L. *et al* (1994) 'Sexual Activity, Contraception and reproductive factors in predicting endometriosis', *American Journal of Epidemiology*, Sep. 15, 140(6): 500–9

Davis K.M. and Rock J.A. 'Endometriosis', *Current Opinins in Obstetrics and Gynaecology*, April 4(2): 229–37

Hill J.A. (1992) 'Immunology and Endometriosis', *Fertility and Sterility*, 58(2): 262–5

Kennedy S. (1993) 'Endometriosis' in MacPherson A. (ed) *Women's Problems in General Practice*, Oxford University Press

O'Connor D.T. (1987) *Endometriosis: Current Reviews in Obstetrics and Gynaecology*, vol. 12, Churchill Livingstone

Olive D.L. (1992) 'Endometriosis: advances in understanding and treatment', *Current Opinions in Obstetrics and Gynaecology*, June 4(3): 380–7

Olive D.L. and Schwartz L.B. (1993) 'Endometriosis', *New England Journal of Medicine*, June 17, 328(24):1759–69

Rock J.A. (1992) 'Pathogenesis of Endometriosis', *Lancet*, Nov. 21, 340; 1264–7

Rock J.A. (1993) 'Endometriosis and Pelvic Pain', *Fertility and Sterility*, Dec. 60(6): 950–1

Shaw R.W. (1992) 'Treatment of Endometriosis', *Lancet*, Nov. 21, 340: 1267–70

Thomas E.J. (1991) 'Endometriosis: Modern Approaches', *Practitioner, 235 (1508): 818–22*

Thomas E.J. (1993) 'Endometriosis: should not be treated because it's there', *British Medical Journal*, Jan. 16, 306(6871): 158–9

Thomas E.J. (1993) 'Endometriosis: still an engima', *British Journal of Obstetrics and Gynaecology*, July 100(7): 615–7

Thomas E.J. and Rock J.A. (eds) (1991) *Modern Approaches to Endometriosis*, Dordrecht; Kluwer Academic

Vessey M.P. *et al* (1993) 'Epidemiology of endometriosis in women attending family planning clinics', *British Medical Journal* Jan. 16, 306(6871): 182–4

Wilson E.A. (ed) (1987) *Endometriosis*, Alan R. Liss Inc, USA (1994) 'An Epidemic Ignored: Endometriosis linked to Dioxin and Immunologic Dysfunction', *Scientific American* April 270 (4): 24–6

USEFUL ADDRESSES

A stamped addressed envelope is welcomed when you make any enquiry.

National Endometriosis Society
Suite 50
Westminster Palace Gardens
1–7 Artillery Row
London SW1P 1RL
0171 222 2776
National Helpline 0171 222 2776
(7–10p.m. daily)

Access to up-to-date information, list of local self-help groups, regular newsletters, workshops etc.

Community Health Council
Look up your local CHC in the phone book for information and advice about your rights in the health service.

Irritable Bowel Syndrome (IBS) Network
St John's House
Hither Green Hospital
Hither Green Lane
London SE13 6RU
0181 698 4611 ext 8194

The Patients Assocation
8 Guilford Street
WC1N 1DT
0171 242 3460
Help with your rights, making complaints etc. Range of leaflets.

PID Network
c/o Women's Health (see below)

CHAPTER 4
SURGICAL TREATMENTS

The Amarant Trust
80 Lambeth Road
London SE1 7PW
0171 401 3855

Association of Chartered
Physiotherapists in Obstetrics
and Gynaecology
Leaflet Secretary
110 Carisbrooke Road
Knighton
Leicester LE2 3PD
Send SAE for leaflet on pelvic
exercises.

Hysterectomy Support Network
3 Lynne Close
Green St Green
Orpington
Kent BR6 6BS
Self-help group meetings,
information and newsletter.

National Osteoporosis Society
Barton Meade House
PO Box 10
Radstock
Bath BA3 3YB
01761 432472
Leaflets and newsletter.

Women's Health (formerly
Women's Health and
Reprodutive Rights Information
Centre)
52–54 Featherstone Street
London EC1Y 8RT
0171 251 6580 (health
enquiries) Supplying
information on a wide range of
issues, maintaining a register of
women's health groups etc.
Send an SAE for publication list
of leaflets; leaflets on tape.

Women's Health Concern
PO Box 1629
London W8 6AU
0171 938 3932
An enquiry service answers
letters and calls; also a
counselling service

CHAPTER 5
ALTERNATIVE APPROACHES

Some of these organisations make a small charge for their information.

British Acupuncture
Association and Register
22 Hockley Road
Rayleigh
Essex S56 8EB
01268 742534

British Naturopathic and
Osteopathic Assocation
6 Netherall Gardens
London NW3 5RR
0171 435 8728
Information and list of
registered practioners.

The Council for Acupuncture
179 Gloucester Place
London NW1 6DX
0171 724 5756

Institute for Complementary
Medicine
PO Box 194
London SE16 1QZ
0171 237 5165
Provides information on
alternative approaches.

International Society of
Professional Aromatherapists
41 Leicester Road
Hinckley
Leicestershire LE10 1LW

British Homoeopathic
Association
27a Devonshire Street
London W1N 1RJ
0171 935 2163
Advice about obtaining
homoeopathy on the NHS.

Community Health Foundation
East-West Centre
London EC1 9EG
0171 251 4076
Programme of courses and
workshops on macrobiotics,
shiatsu etc.

Dr Edward Bach Centre
Mount Vernon
Sotwell
Wallingford
Oxon OX10 0PZ
01491 34678
General information, order
form for remedies and booklist.

International Federation of
Aromatherapists
4 East Mearn Road
Dulwich
London SE21 8HA

National Institute of Medical
Herbalists Ltd
9 Palace Gate
Exeter EX1 1JA
01392 426022

Positive Health Centre
101 Harley Street
London W1
0171 935 1811
Courses in autogenic training
(amongst others).

The Society of Homoeopaths
2 Artizan Road
Northampton
NN1 4HU
01604 21400
List of homoeopaths who are
not doctors (and therefore
cannot practise on the NHS).
Information on homoeopathy in
pregnancy and childbirth.

Register of Traditional Chinese
Medicine
19 Trinity Road
London N2 8JJ
0181 883 8431

The Traditional Acupuncture
Society
1 The Ridgeway
Stratford-upon-Avon
Warwickshire CV37 9JL
01789 298798

CHAPTER 6
ENDOMETRIOSIS AND INFERTILITY

Adoption Project, Thomas
Coram Foundation for Children
40 Brunswick Square
London WC1N 1AZ
0171 278 2424

Child
P.O. Box 154
Hounslow
Middlesex TW5 0EZ
0181 571 4367
Information and counselling
service for members. Fund-
raising for research into the
causes of infertility.

British Agencies for Adoption
and Fostering (BAAF)
11 Southwark Street
London SE1 1RQ
0171 407 8800

Family Planning Information
Service
27–29 Mortimer Street
London W1N 7RJ
0171 636 7866
Register of infertility services.

ISSUE (The National Fertility
Association)
509 Aldridge Road
Great Barr
Birmingham B44 8NA
0121 344 4414
Large organisation offering
information and counselling.
Find out about your regional
group.

ISSUE (Scotland)
21 Castle Street
Edinburgh EH2 3DN
0131 225 2464

National Foster Care
Association (NFCA)
Leonard House
5–7 Marshalsea Road
London SE1 1EP
0171 828 6266

Parents for Children
41 Southgate Road
London N1 3JP
0171 359 7530

Parent to Parent Information &
Adoption Service (PPIAS)
Lower Boddington
Daventry
Northants
NN11 6YB
01327 60295
A support and information
service for families who have or
are planning to adopt.

CHAPTER 7
ENDOMETRIOSIS AND PREGNANCY

Association for the
Improvement in Maternity
Services
40 Kingswood Avenue
London NW6 6LS
0181 960 5585

Assocation for Post-Natal
Illness
25 Jerdan Place
London SW6 1BE
0171 386 0868

Cry-sis Support Group
BM Crysis
London WC1N 3XX
0171 404 5011 (Helpline)
Self-help with crying babies.
National network of groups.

Meet-a-Mum Association
14 Willis Road
Croydon CR0 2XX
0181 665 0357

National Childbirth Trust
(NCT)
Alexandra House
Oldham Terrace
Acton
London W3 6NH
0181 992 8637

Foresight
28 The Paddock
Godalming
Surrey GU7 1XD
01483 427839

The Miscarriage Association
c/o Clayton Hospital
Northgate
Wakefield
WF1 3JS
01924 200 799

Stillbirth and Neonatal Death
Society (SANDS)
28 Portland Place
London W1N 4DE
0171 436 5881 (Helpline)

CHAPTER 8
UNDERSTANDING YOUR FEELINGS

British Association for
Counselling
1 Regent Place
Rugby CV21 2PJ
01788 550899
Advice about local counsellors,
including those who specialise
in sexual problems.

MIND (National Association
for Mental Health)
Granta House
15–19 Broadway
Stratford
London E15 4BQ
0181 519 2122
Look in the phone book for
your local association.

Institute of Psychosexual
Medicine
11 Chandos Street
London W1M 9DE
0171 580 0631

RELATE – National Marriage
Guidance
Herbert Gray College
Little Church Street
Rugby
Warwicks. CV21 3AP
01788 573241/560811
Look up your local branch in
the phone book.

Westminster Pastoral
Foundation
23 Kensington Square
London W8 5HN
0171 937 6956
Lists counsellors who can
attend to spiritual needs.

Women's Therapy Centre
6–9 Manor Gardens
London N7 6LA
0171 263 6200 (advice and
information line)
Offer therapists, courses and
workshops.

CHAPTER 9
GETTING TO GRIPS WITH PAIN

See page 165 for addresses of societies dealing with alternative therapies.

College of Health
St Margaret's House
21 Old Ford Road
London E2 9PL
0181 983 1225
A range of relevant publications
for purchase including a
directory of pain clinics.

Neen Pain Management
Systems
Barn Lodge
Gooseberry Hill
Swanton Morley
Dereham
Norfolk NR20 4NR
01362 698966
Can supply a small and easy-to-
use TENS machine if you
cannot find a local supplier.

Pain Wise (UK)
33 Kingsdown Park
Tankerton
Kent CT5 2DT
01227 277886 (after 2 p.m.)
Advice and information on pain
management programmes.

ENDOMETRIOSIS IN CYBERSPACE

If you want to participate in discussions about endometriosis on the Internet you will need a computer with a modem (link through a telephone line) and a subscription to what is known as an Internet service provider which will give you an e-mail address on the Internet. Services like Compuserve can also give you the type of access you need (but may be more expensive).

Advice on how to establish the technical link and subscribe is available from a variety of sources. For example, there are numerous of books on the Internet – try your library or bookshop. Many modems are sold with free, introductory membership of Compuserve or another Internet service provider so computer sales people can often help. It is also worth asking your local library if it offers Internet access or advice and invetigating what is available at your local college. People have been known to enrol for a single class simply to get a free internet address! However, you may feel you need the class as well!

Depending on your technical skills, connecting to the Internet can be rather tricky and even frustrating, but it is getting easier as the service providers start to improve access. Using the Internet isn't difficult once your connection is established so it is worth getting that initial help if you need it.

Once you're on the Internet there are various types of discussion groups and sources of information. WITSENDO is a group dedicated to the discussion of endometriosis. The group is only available to its subscribers and the discussions are checked by a moderator (ie. someone who voluntarily checks all the messages for obscenities, libel, etc., before releasing them onto the Internet). If you want to receive and participate in WITSENDO (and become known as a WIT-SENDER!), send an e-mail message as follows:

To: listserv@listserv.dartmouth.edu
Subject: [can be left empty]
Message: SUBSCRIBE WITSENDO firstname lastname [where firstname and lastname are your own].

The listserv address is only used for subscribing and administrative functions such as retrieving archives of old messages. You will automatically receive back a set of instructions on how to use WITSENDO. To contribute a message to WITSENDO send it to a different address:

To: WITSENDO@DARTMOUTH.EDU
Subject: Topic of your message
Message: What you want to say

You will get an automatic acknowledgement message back from the Dartmouth computer almost immediately. Your message will appear later as an e-mail to all the WITSENDO subscribers when the moderator releases a batch of messages.

The access information above was kindly provided by Imogen Bertin in Ireland who has offered to help anyone who wishes to use WITSENDO. Her e-mail address is imogen@ctc.ie and her international telephone number is 00353 21 887300.

If you have World Wide Web access on the Internet, Dr Mark Perloe operates a WWW site about endometriosis at:

http://www.mindspring.com/~mperloe

Endometriosis has also been discussed in various Usenet Newsgroups (for examples, see below). These groups do not charge a subscription but are more public so you may not want to discuss personal and intimate details in these groups.

soc.women
sci.med
sci.med.pharmacy
alt.health
alt.folklore.herbs
alt.sexual.abuse.recovery

INDEX

Page numbers in *italic* refer to the illustrations

Other Positive Parenting titles available from
VERMILION

To order any of these books direct from Vermilion (p+p free), use the form below or call our credit-card hotline on **01279 427203.**

Please send me

...... copies of **ALTERNATIVE MATERNITY** @ £8.99 each

...... copies of **HOME BIRTH** @ £8.99 each

...... copies of **PLANNING A BABY?** @ £8.99 each

...... copies of **CHOOSING OLDER MOTHERHOOD** @ £8.99

...... copies of **YOUR NEW BABY** @ £8.99 each

Mr/Ms/Mrs/Miss/Other (BlockLetters)

....

Address...

....

....

Postcode...........................Signed.................................

HOW TO PAY

☐ I enclose a cheque/postal order for

£.............................. made payable to 'Vermilion'

☐ I wish to pay by Access/Visa card (delete where appropriate)

Card Number ☐☐☐☐☐☐☐☐☐☐☐☐☐☐☐☐

Expiry Date ☐☐☐☐

Post order to **Murlyn Services Ltd, PO Box 50, Harlow, Essex CM17 ODZ.**

POSTAGE AND PACKING ARE FREE. Offer open in Great Britain including Northern Ireland. Books should arrive less than 28 days after we receive your order; they are subject to availability at time of ordering. If not entirely satisfied return in the same packaging and condition as received with a covering letter within 7 days. Vermilion books are available from all good booksellers.